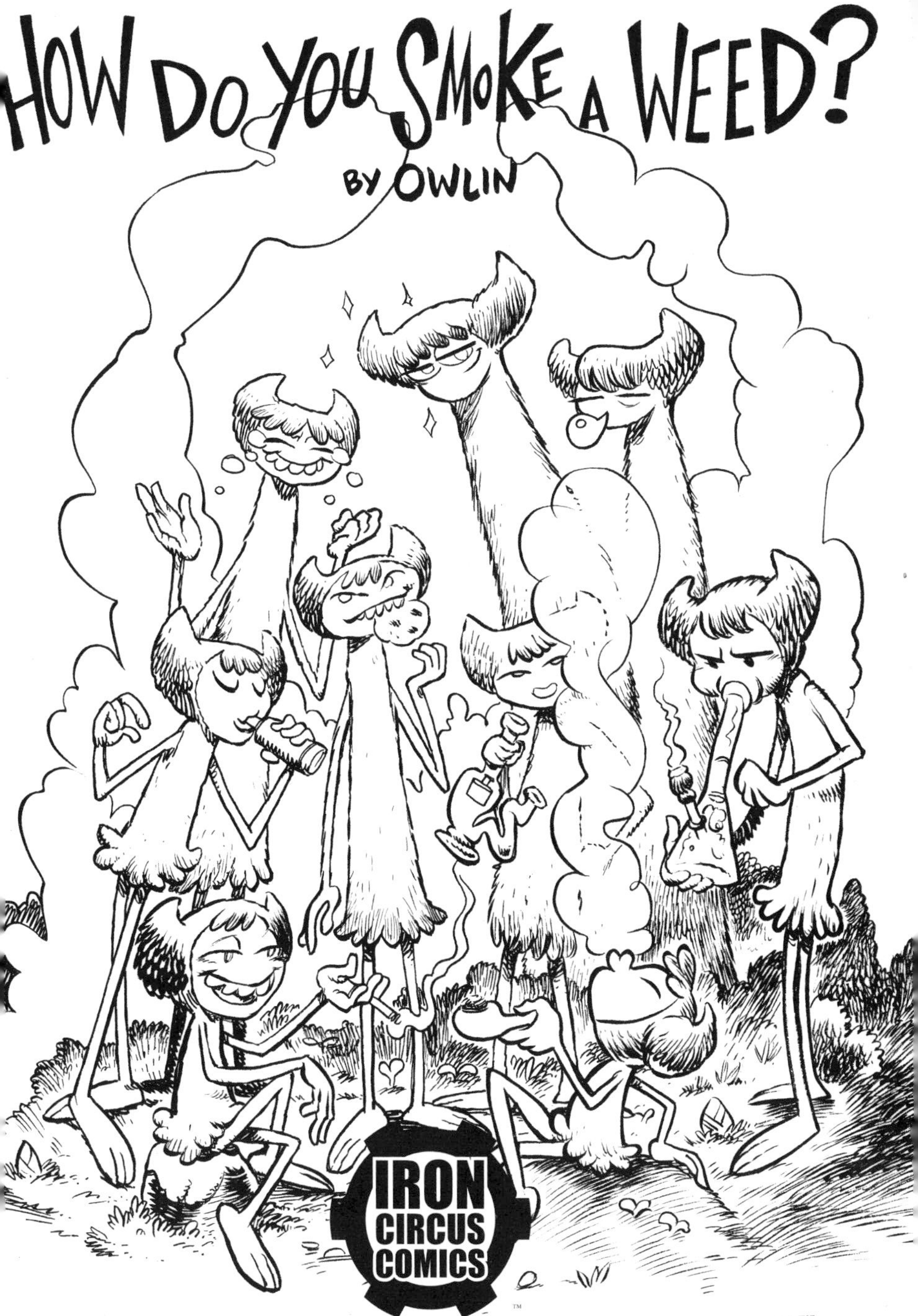
HOW DO YOU SMOKE A WEED?
BY OWLIN
IRON CIRCUS COMICS

trange and g

nquiry@ironcircus.com www.ironcircus.com

creators
Lin Visel, Joseph Bergin III, and Lauren Keller

publisher, editor
C. Spike Trotman

book designer
Matt Sheridan

proofreader
Abby Lehrke

print technician
Rhiannon Rasmussen-Silverstein

published by
Iron Circus Comics
329 West 18th Street, Suite 604
Chicago, IL 60616
ironcircus.com

first edition: February 2019

print book ISBN: 978-1-945820-16-8

10 9 8 7 6 5 4 3 2 1

HOW DO YOU SMOKE A WEED?

Names: Owlin. | Keller, Lauren (Lauren Nicole) | Visel, Lin. | Bergin, Joseph, III.
Title: How do you smoke a weed? / by Owlin ... with assistance from Lauren Keller, Lin Visel, a
    Joseph Bergin III.
Description: [Chicago, Illinois] : Iron Circus Comics, [2018] | "A comics guide to a responsib
    high."--Cover.
Identifiers: ISBN 9781945820168
Subjects: LCSH: Marijuana--Comic books, strips, etc. | Smoking--Study and teaching--Com
    books, strips, etc. | LCGFT: Fantasy fiction. | Graphic novels.
Classification: LCC PN6727.O95 H69 2018 | DDC 741.5973 [Fic]--dc23

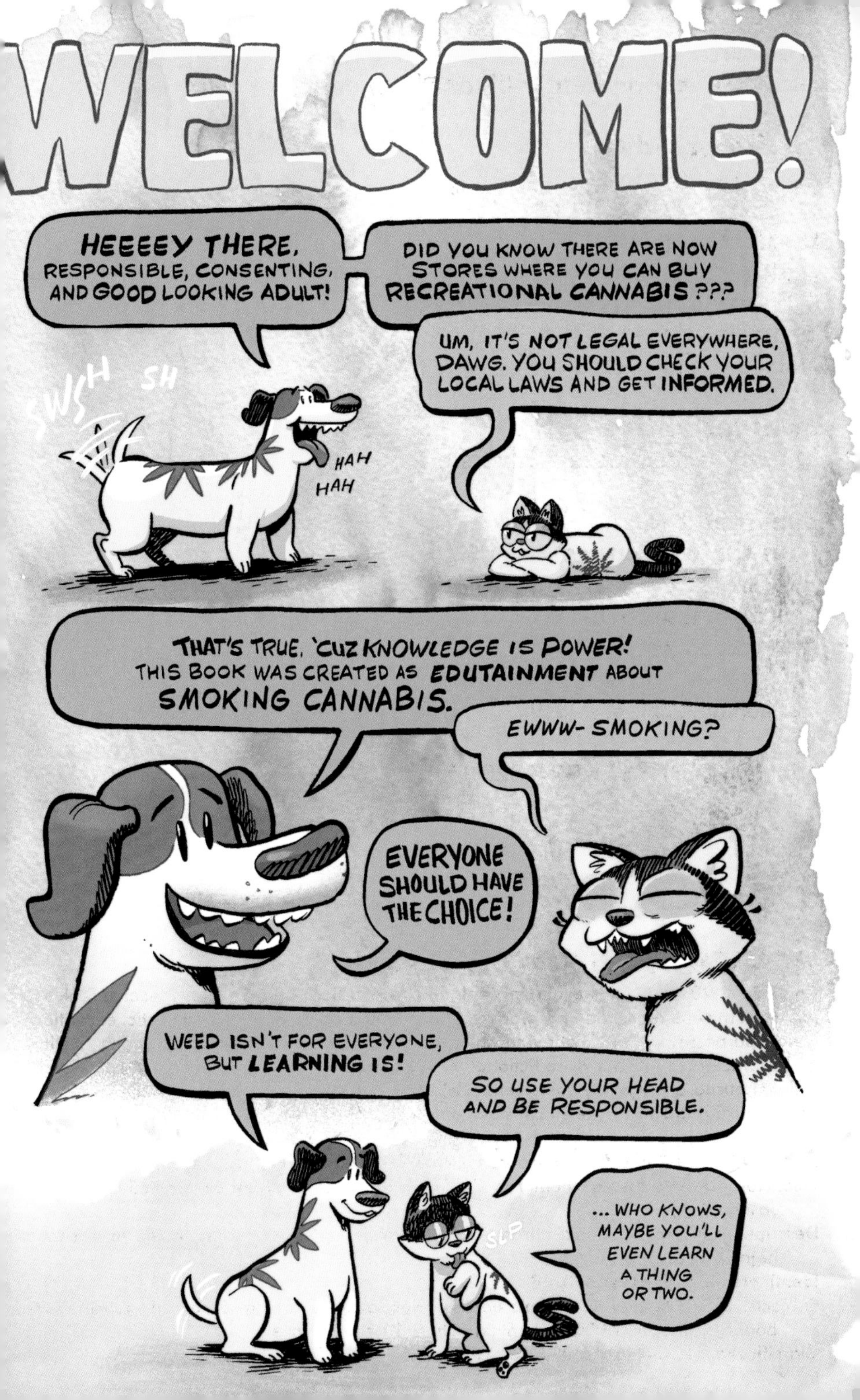
WELCOME!
HEEEEY THERE, RESPONSIBLE, CONSENTING, AND GOOD LOOKING ADULT!
DID YOU KNOW THERE ARE NOW STORES WHERE YOU CAN BUY RECREATIONAL CANNABIS???
UM, IT'S NOT LEGAL EVERYWHERE, DAWG. YOU SHOULD CHECK YOUR LOCAL LAWS AND GET INFORMED.
SWSH SH
HAH HAH
THAT'S TRUE. 'CUZ KNOWLEDGE IS POWER! THIS BOOK WAS CREATED AS EDUTAINMENT ABOUT SMOKING CANNABIS.
EWWW- SMOKING?
EVERYONE SHOULD HAVE THE CHOICE!
WEED ISN'T FOR EVERYONE, BUT LEARNING IS!
SO USE YOUR HEAD AND BE RESPONSIBLE.
SLP
... WHO KNOWS, MAYBE YOU'LL EVEN LEARN A THING OR TWO.

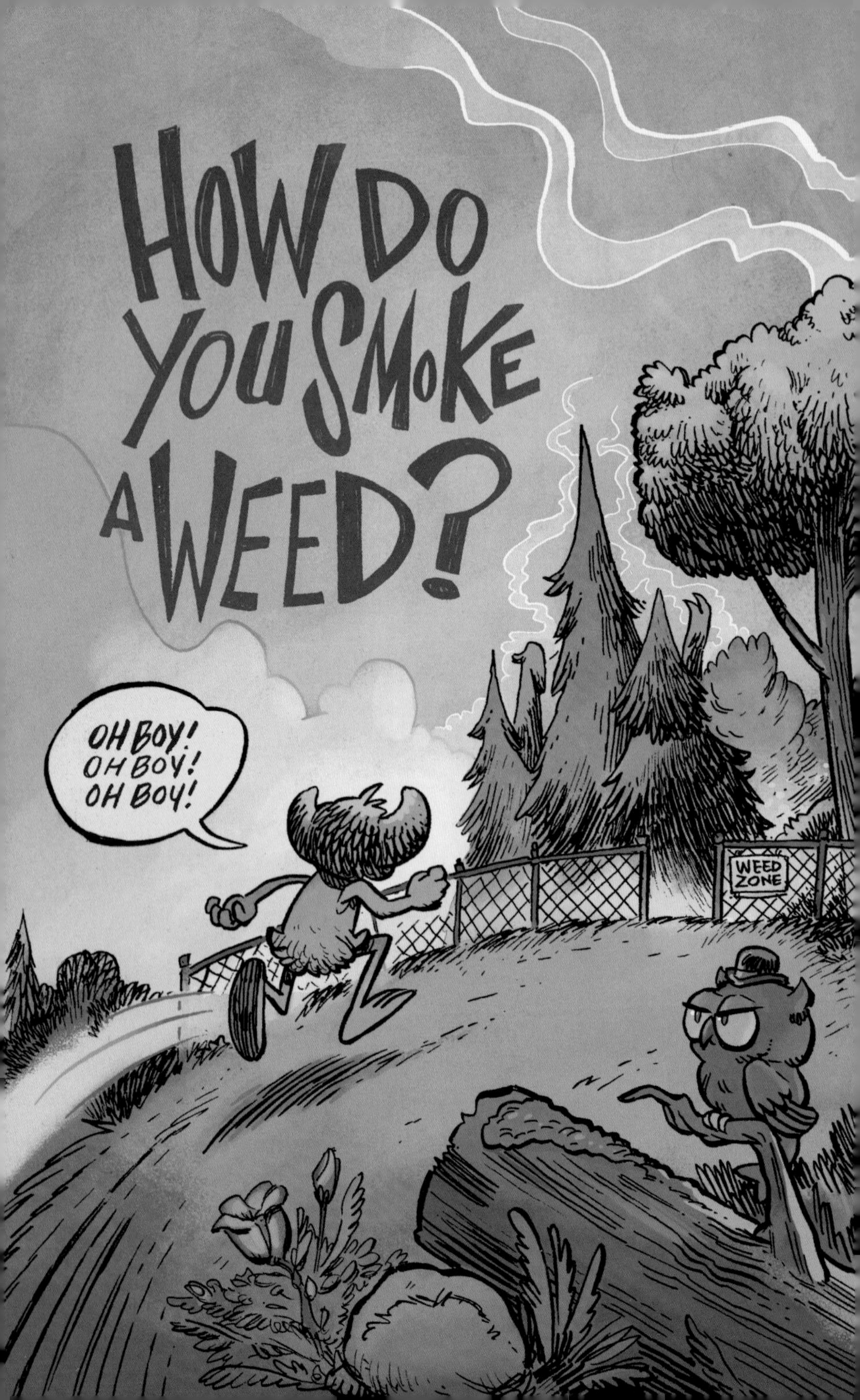
HOW DO YOU SMOKE A WEED?
OH BOY! OH BOY! OH BOY!
WEED ZONE

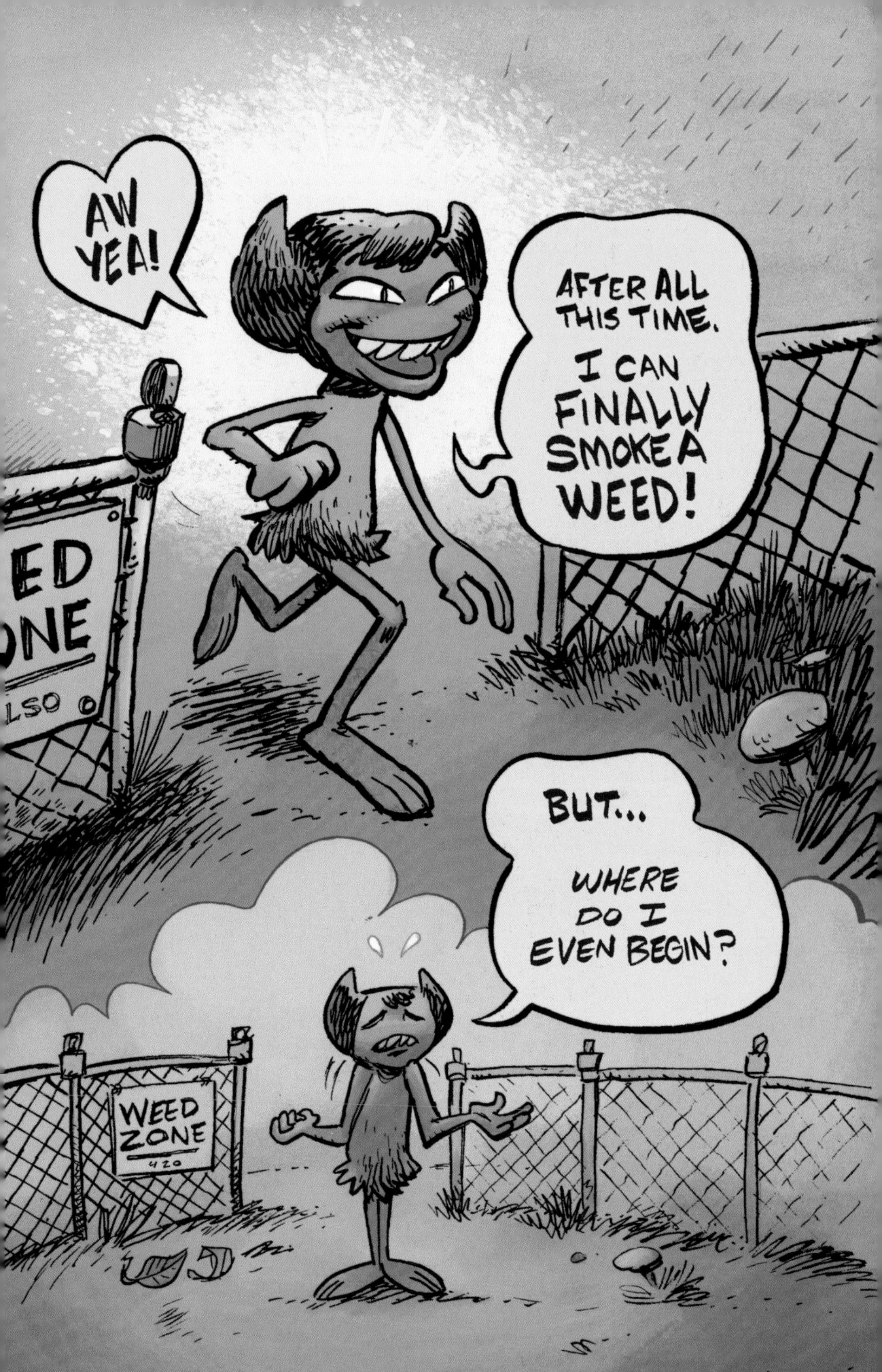
AW YEA!
AFTER ALL THIS TIME.
I CAN FINALLY SMOKE A WEED!
ED
ONE
LSO
BUT...
WHERE DO I EVEN BEGIN?
WEED ZONE
420

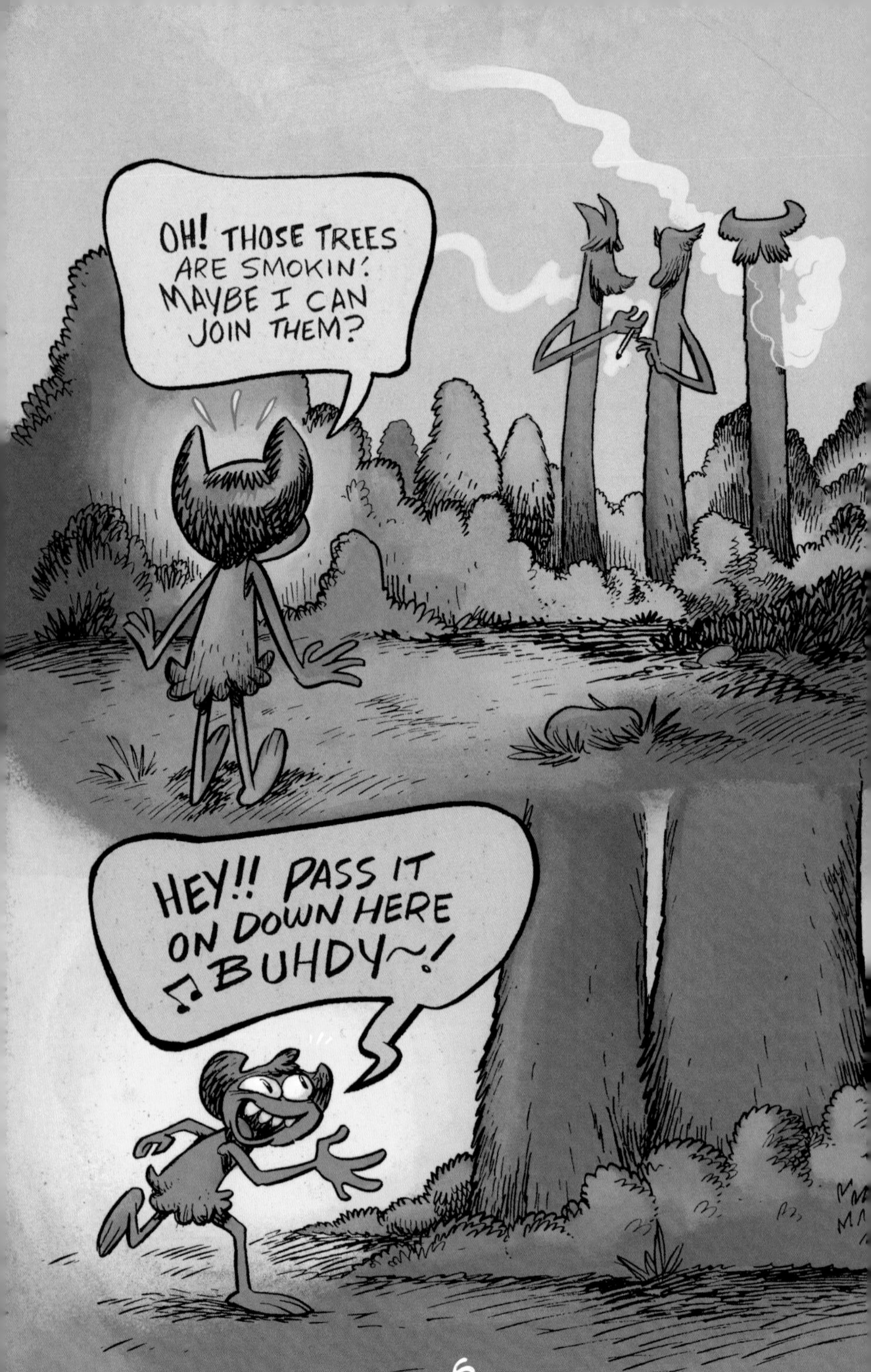
OH! THOSE TREES ARE SMOKIN'! MAYBE I CAN JOIN THEM?
HEY!! PASS IT ON DOWN HERE ♫BUHDY~!

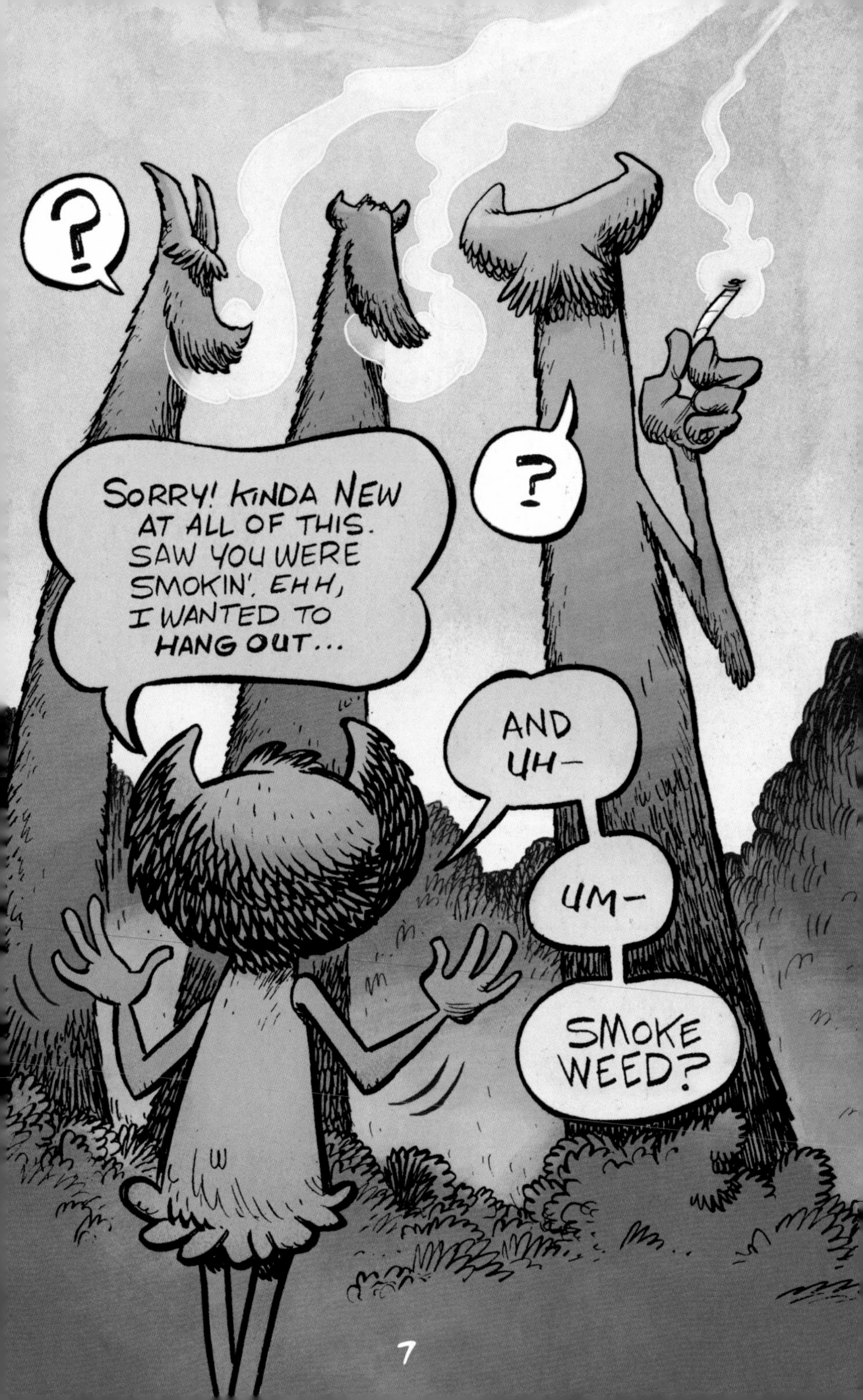
?
SORRY! KINDA NEW AT ALL OF THIS. SAW YOU WERE SMOKIN'. EHH, I WANTED TO HANG OUT...
?
AND UH-
UM-
SMOKE WEED?

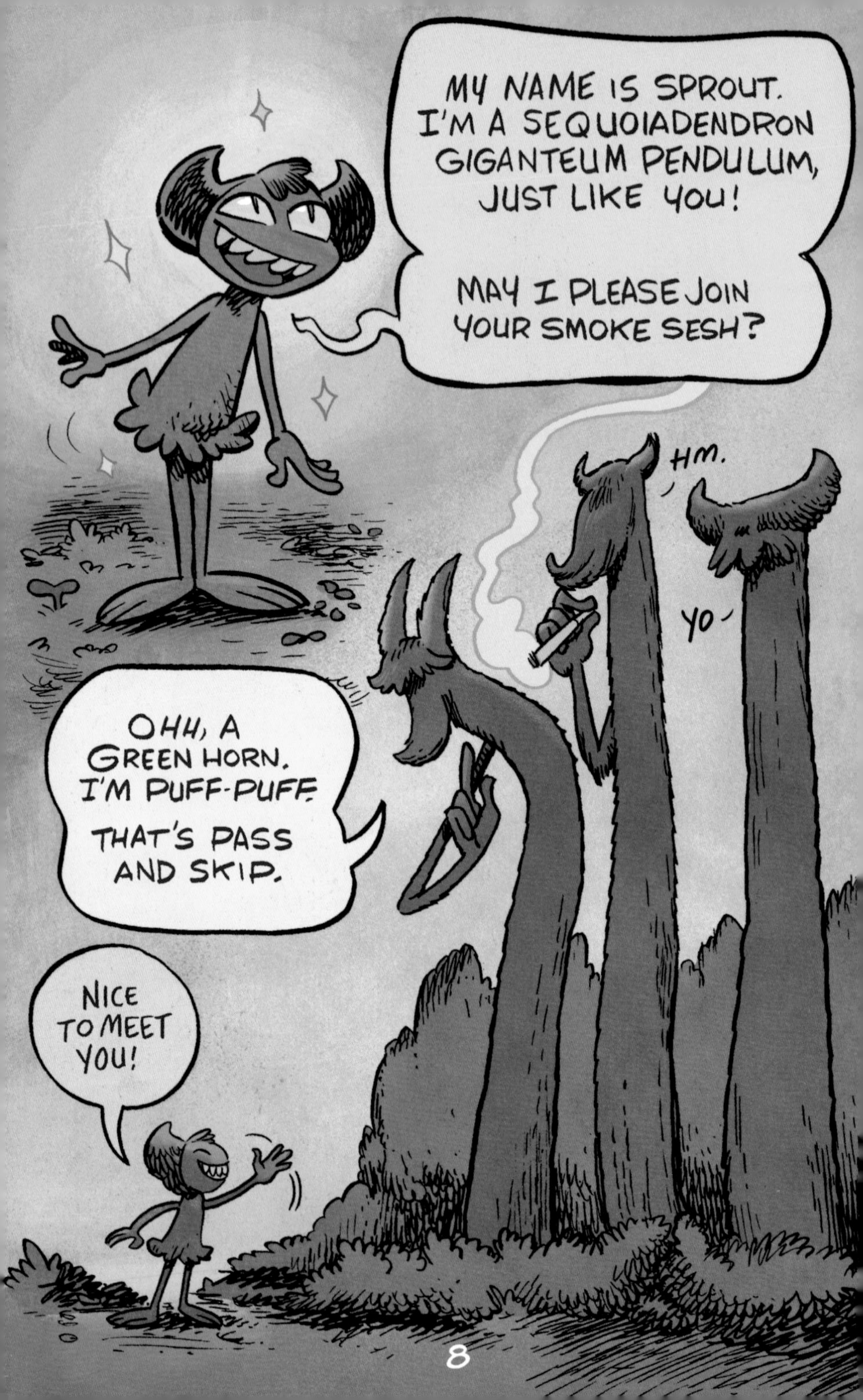

MY NAME IS SPROUT. I'M A SEQUOIADENDRON GIGANTEUM PENDULUM, JUST LIKE YOU!
MAY I PLEASE JOIN YOUR SMOKE SESH?
HM.
YO-
OHH, A GREEN HORN. I'M PUFF-PUFF.
THAT'S PASS AND SKIP.
NICE TO MEET YOU!

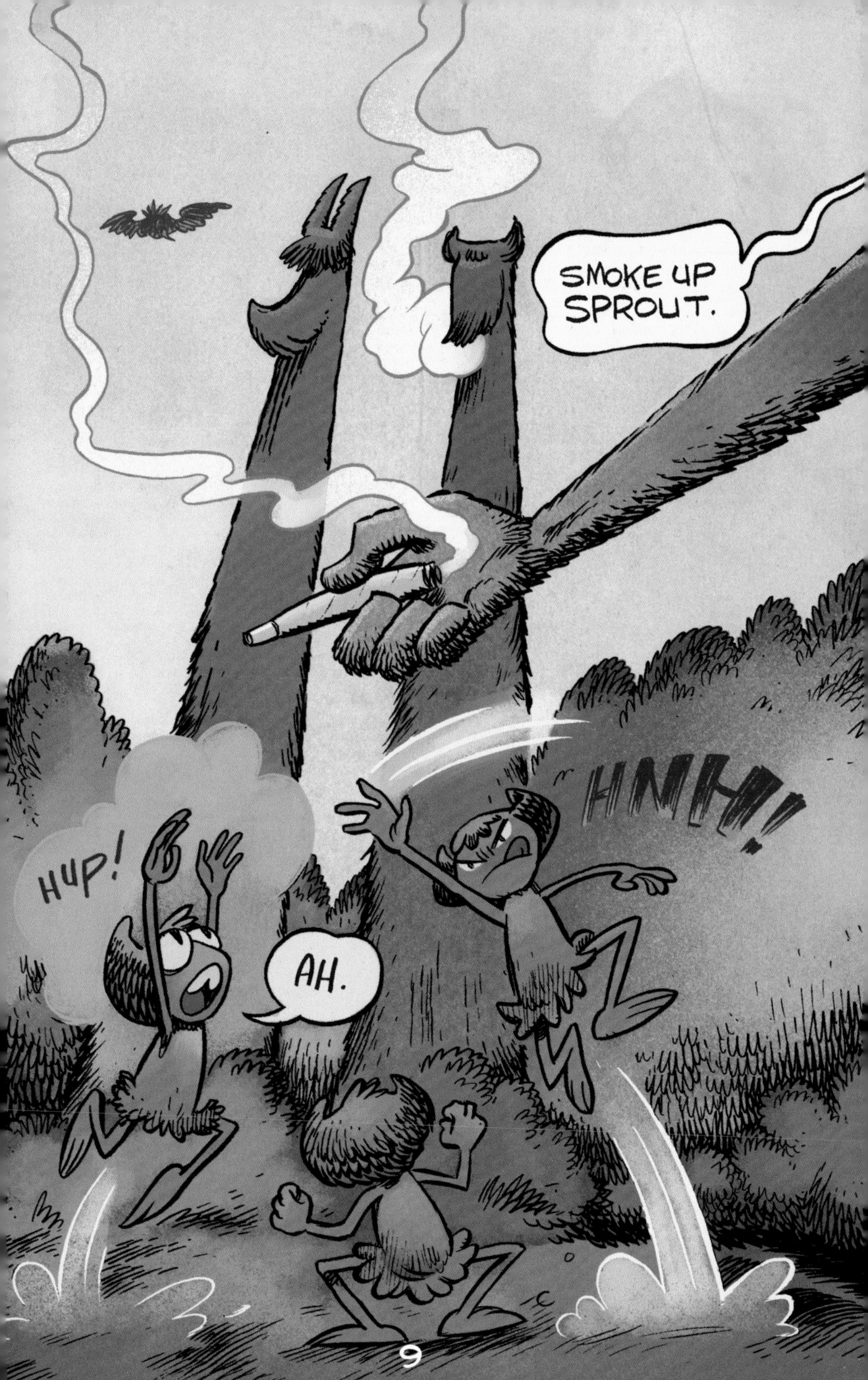
SMOKE UP SPROUT.
HNH!!
HUP!
AH.

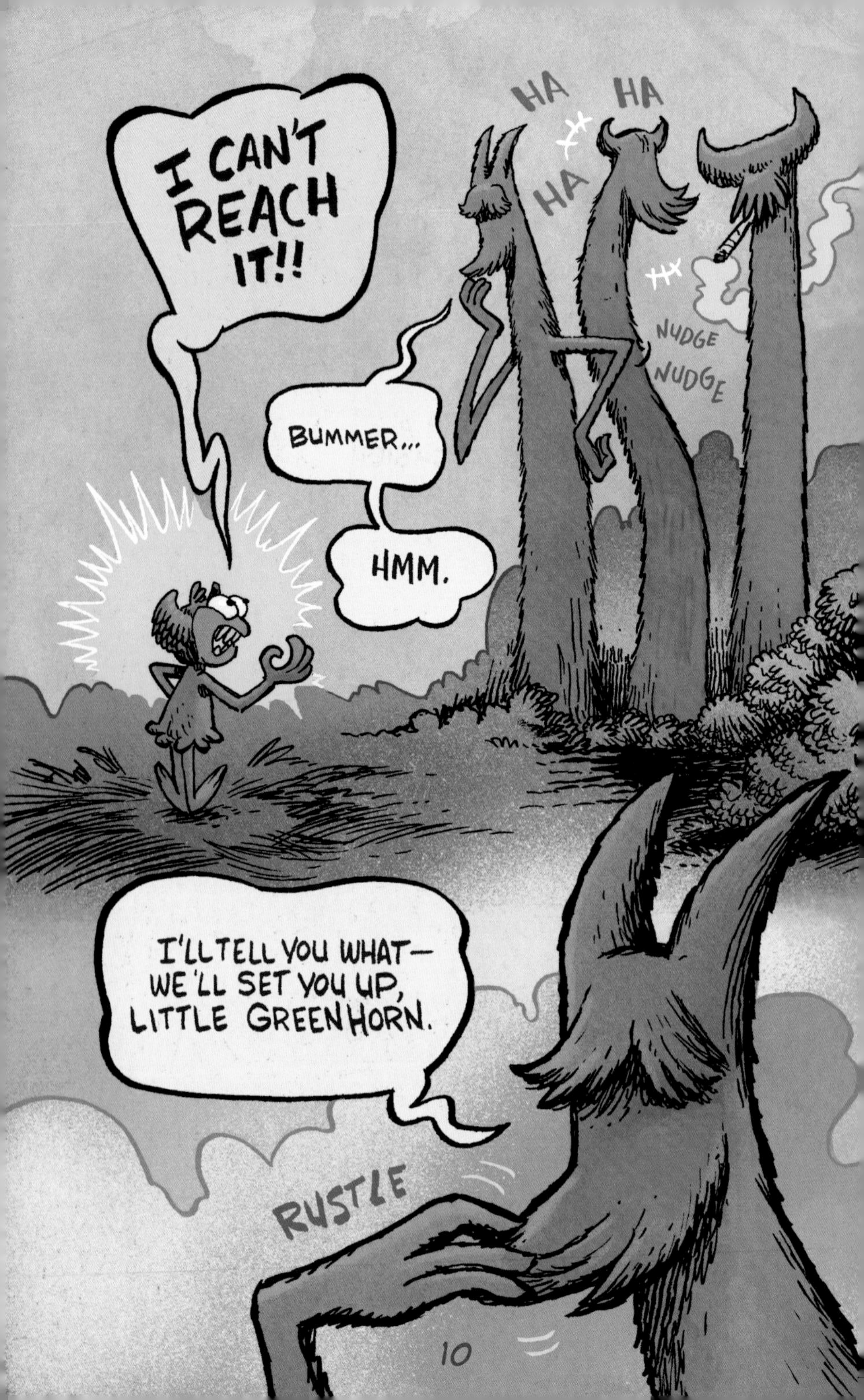
I CAN'T REACH IT!!
HA HA
HA
BUMMER...
HMM.
NUDGE
NUDGE
I'LL TELL YOU WHAT— WE'LL SET YOU UP, LITTLE GREENHORN.
RUSTLE

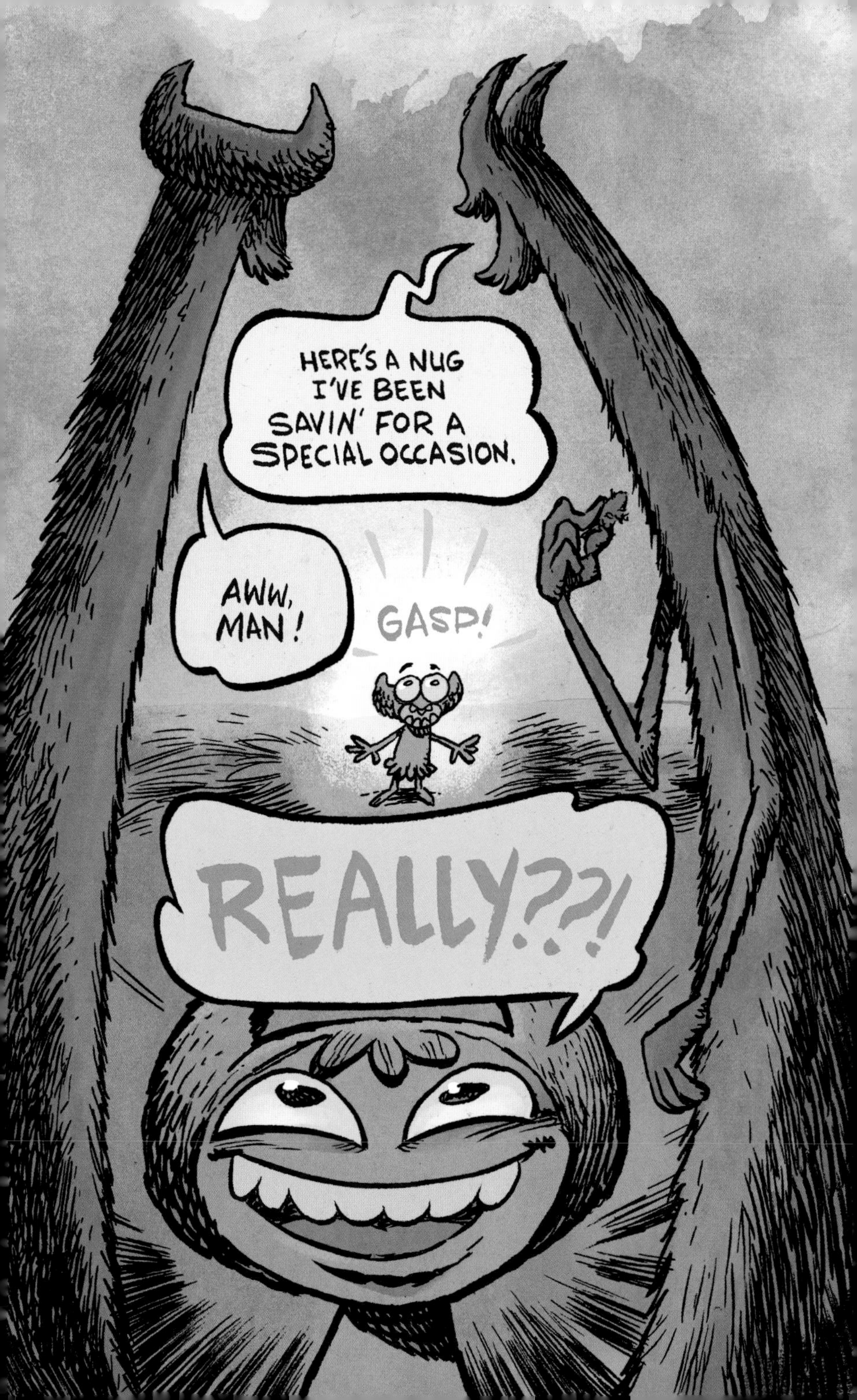
HERE'S A NUG I'VE BEEN SAVIN' FOR A SPECIAL OCCASION.
AWW, MAN!
GASP!
REALLY??!

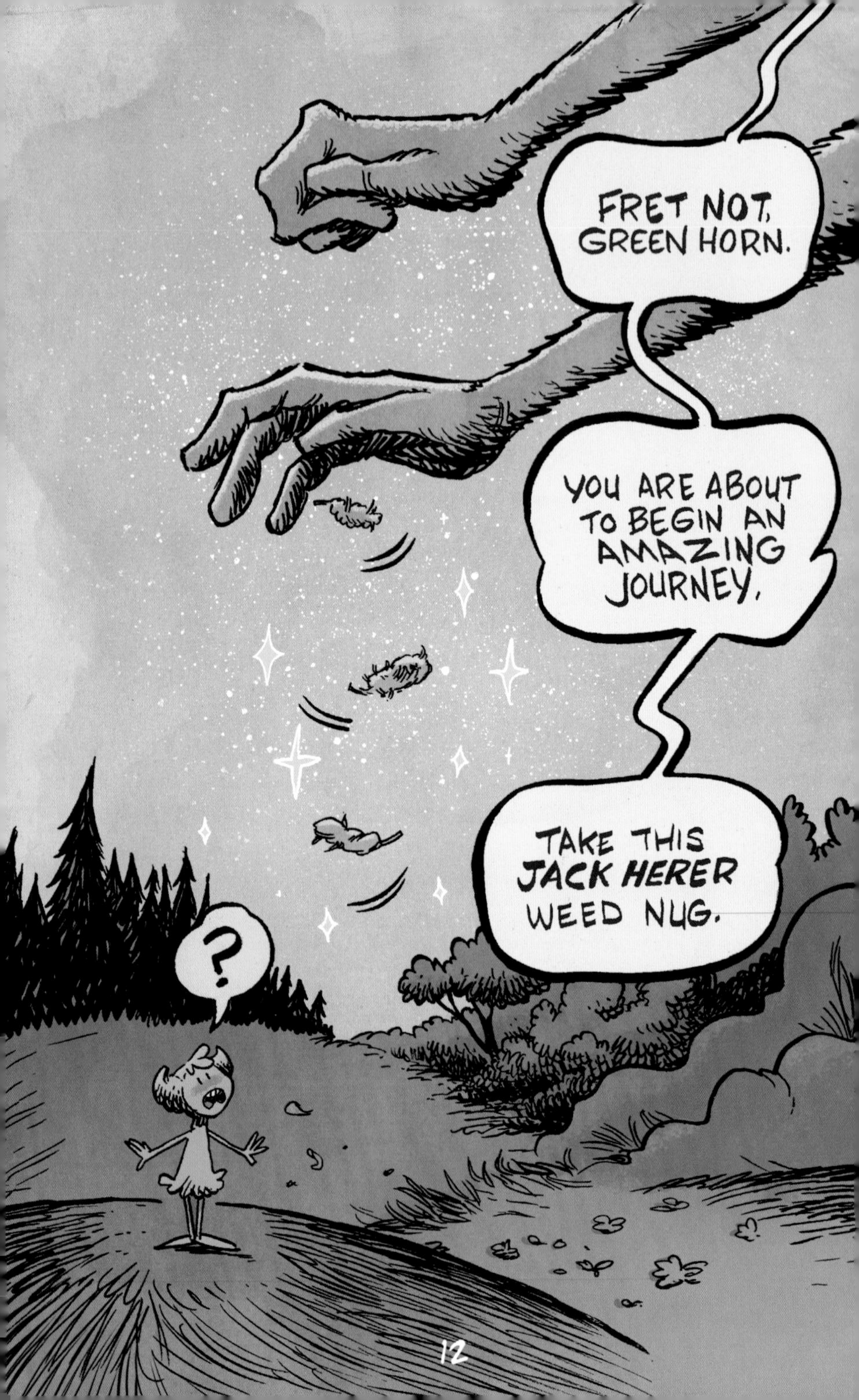
FRET NOT, GREEN HORN.
YOU ARE ABOUT TO BEGIN AN AMAZING JOURNEY.
TAKE THIS JACK HERER WEED NUG.
?

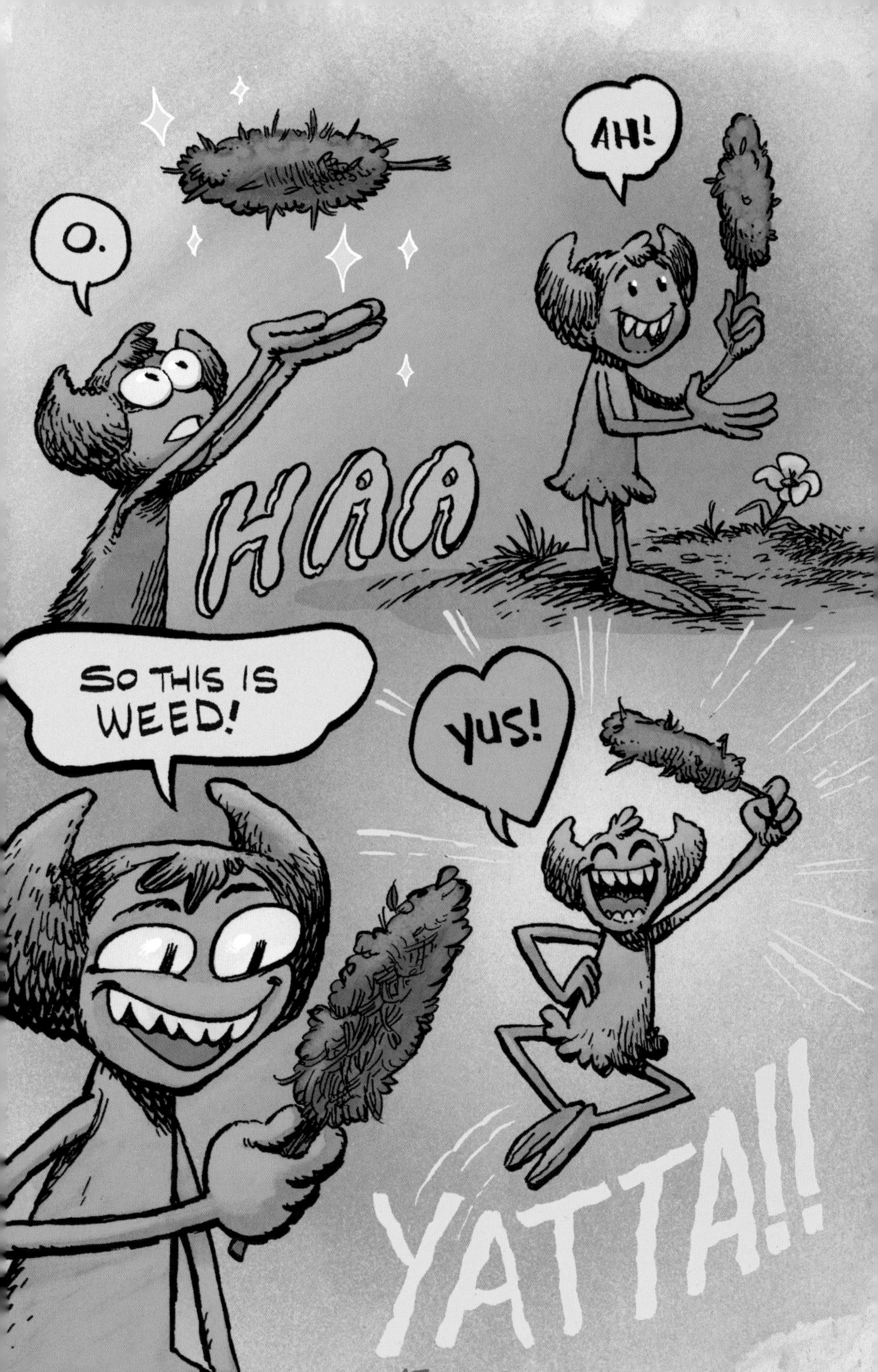
O.
AH!
HAA
SO THIS IS WEED!
yus!
YATTA!!

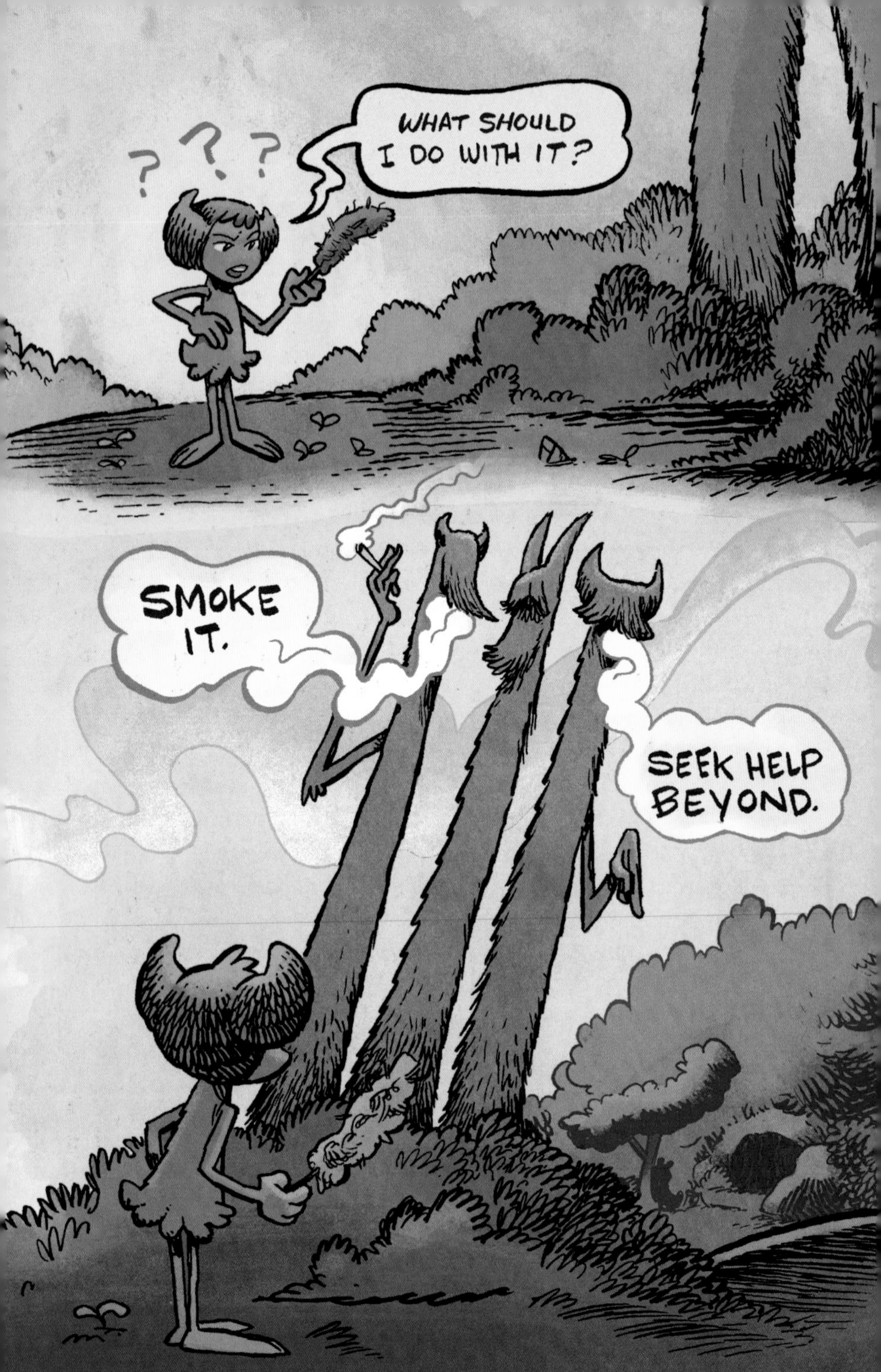
? ? ?
WHAT SHOULD I DO WITH IT?
SMOKE IT.
SEEK HELP BEYOND.

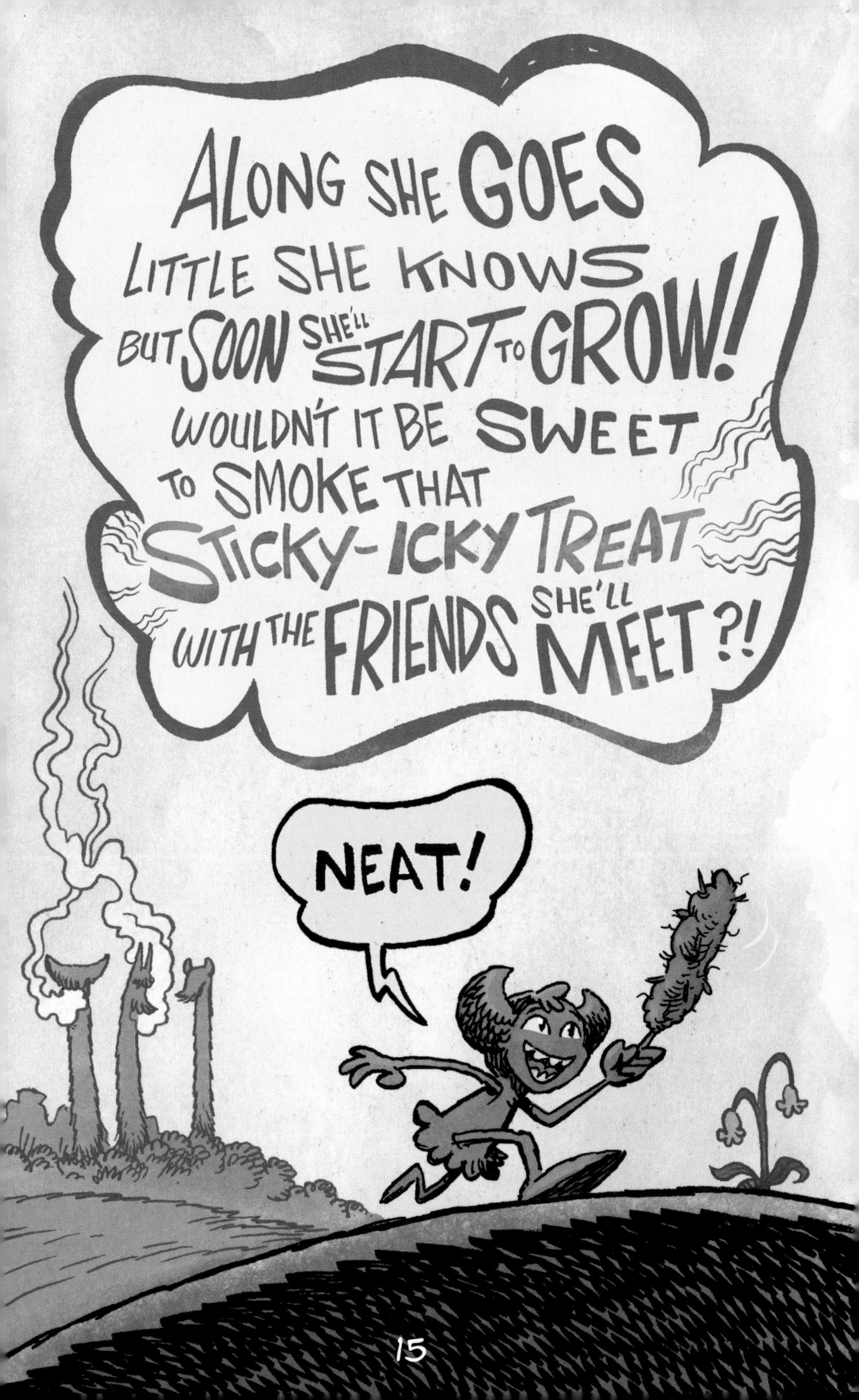
ALONG SHE GOES
LITTLE SHE KNOWS
BUT SOON SHE'LL START TO GROW!
WOULDN'T IT BE SWEET
TO SMOKE THAT
STICKY-ICKY TREAT
WITH THE FRIENDS SHE'LL MEET?!
NEAT!

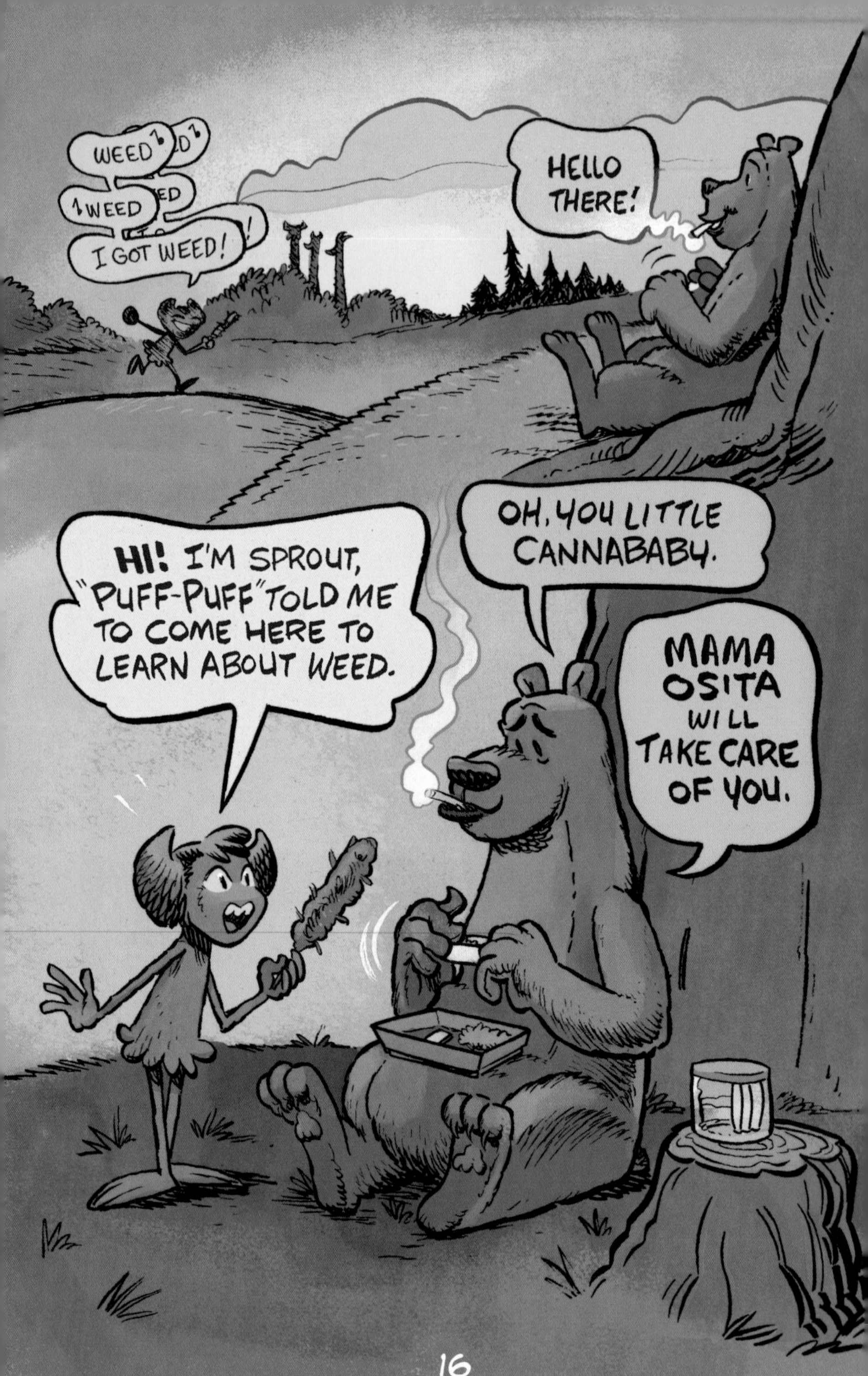
WEED
WEED
I GOT WEED!
HELLO THERE!
HI! I'M SPROUT, "PUFF-PUFF" TOLD ME TO COME HERE TO LEARN ABOUT WEED.
OH, YOU LITTLE CANNABABY.
MAMA OSITA WILL TAKE CARE OF YOU.

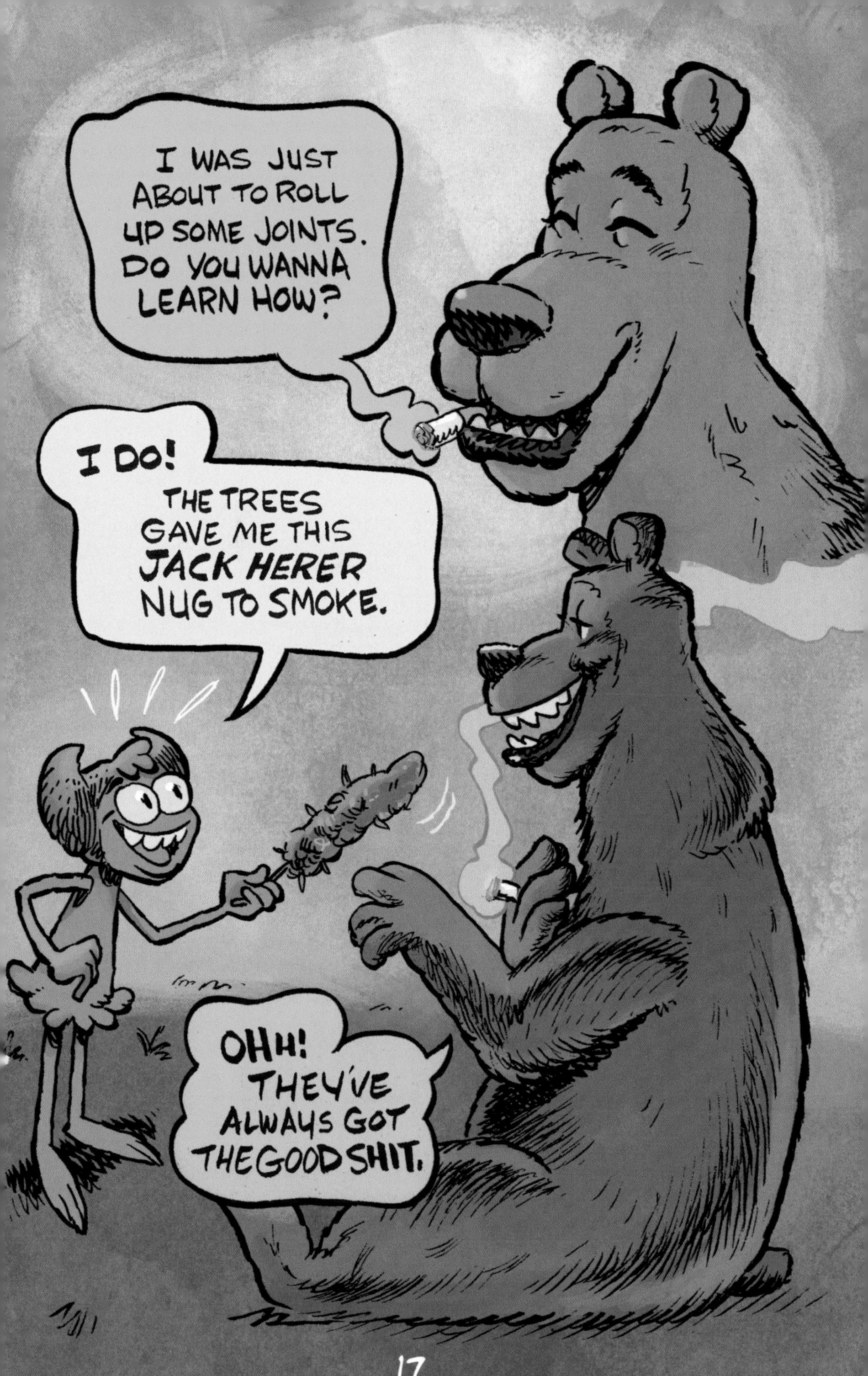
I WAS JUST ABOUT TO ROLL UP SOME JOINTS. DO YOU WANNA LEARN HOW?
I DO!
THE TREES GAVE ME THIS JACK HERER NUG TO SMOKE.
OHH! THEY'VE ALWAYS GOT THE GOOD SHIT.

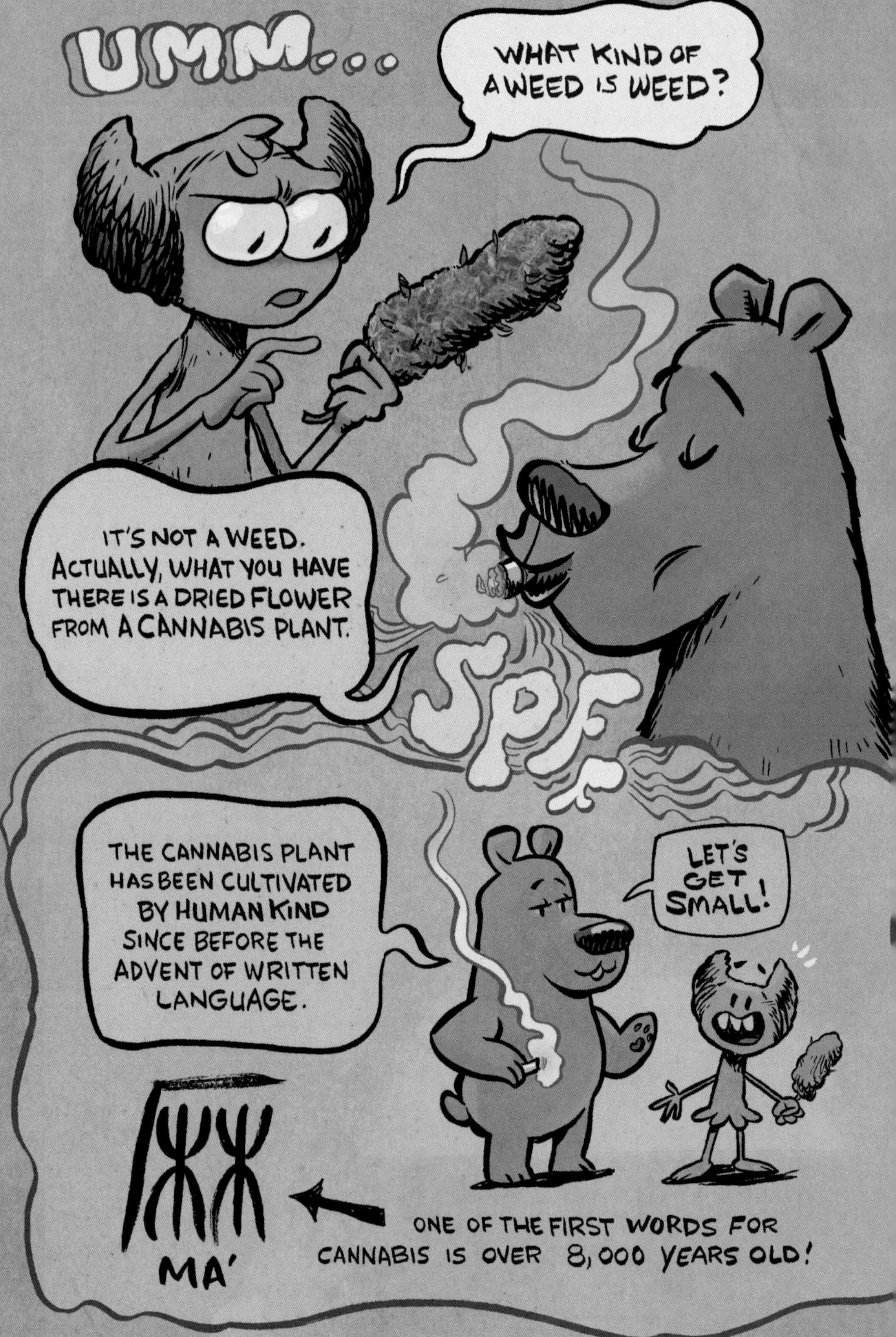
UMM...
WHAT KIND OF A WEED IS WEED?
IT'S NOT A WEED. ACTUALLY, WHAT YOU HAVE THERE IS A DRIED FLOWER FROM A CANNABIS PLANT.
SPF
THE CANNABIS PLANT HAS BEEN CULTIVATED BY HUMAN KIND SINCE BEFORE THE ADVENT OF WRITTEN LANGUAGE.
LET'S GET SMALL!
MA'
ONE OF THE FIRST WORDS FOR CANNABIS IS OVER 8,000 YEARS OLD!

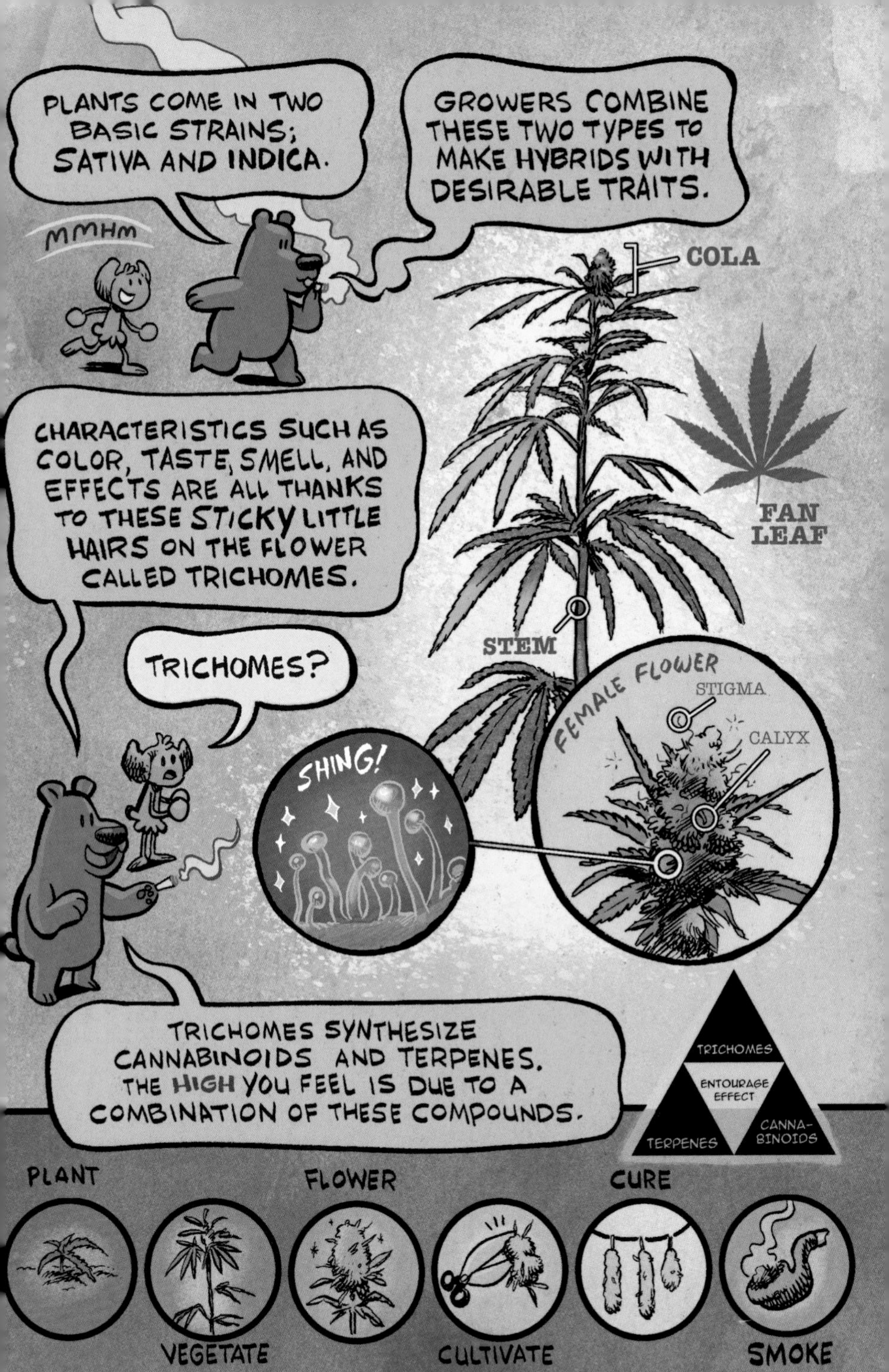
PLANTS COME IN TWO BASIC STRAINS; SATIVA AND INDICA.
MMHM
GROWERS COMBINE THESE TWO TYPES TO MAKE HYBRIDS WITH DESIRABLE TRAITS.
COLA
FAN LEAF
CHARACTERISTICS SUCH AS COLOR, TASTE, SMELL, AND EFFECTS ARE ALL THANKS TO THESE STICKY LITTLE HAIRS ON THE FLOWER CALLED TRICHOMES.
STEM
TRICHOMES?
FEMALE FLOWER
STIGMA
CALYX
SHING!
TRICHOMES SYNTHESIZE CANNABINOIDS AND TERPENES. THE HIGH YOU FEEL IS DUE TO A COMBINATION OF THESE COMPOUNDS.
TRICHOMES
ENTOURAGE EFFECT
TERPENES
CANNA-BINOIDS
PLANT
VEGETATE
FLOWER
CULTIVATE
CURE
SMOKE

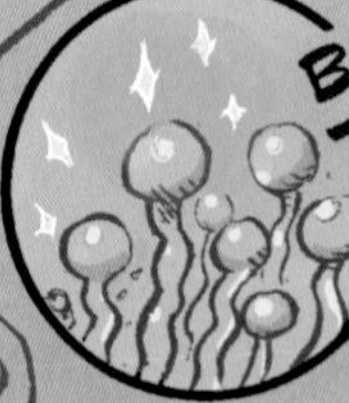

BORN OF TRICHOMES

SMELLS GOOD IN HERE...

 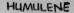

TERPENES!

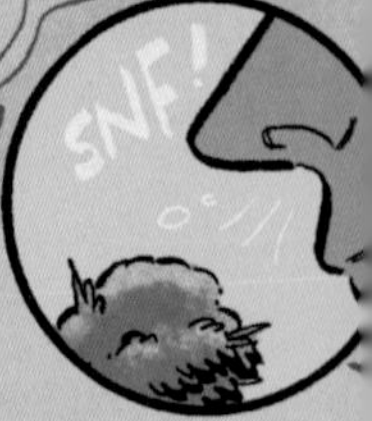

THESE GIVE EACH INDIVIDUAL STRAIN ITS AROMA AND EFFECTS. HERE ARE THE SIX MOST COMMON TERPENES.

CARYOPHYLLENE

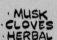

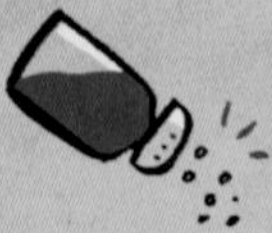

- PEPPER
- WOOD
- SPICE

HUMULENE

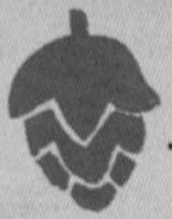

- WOODY
- EARTHY
- HOPS-LIKE

PINENE

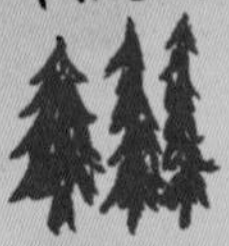

- SHARP
- SWEET
- PINE

MYRCENE

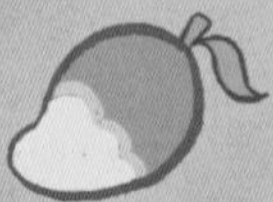

- MUSK
- CLOVES
- HERBAL
- CITRUS

LINALOOL

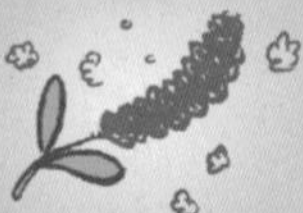

- FLORAL
- CITRUS
- SPICE

LIMONENE

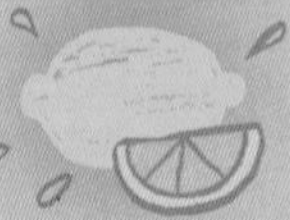

- CITRUS
- LEMON
- ORANGE

THEY WORK AS A NATURAL DEFENSE SYSTEM FOR THE PLANT.

THEY'RE ALSO THE BUILDING BLOCKS FOR **THC** AND OTHER CANNABINOIDS.

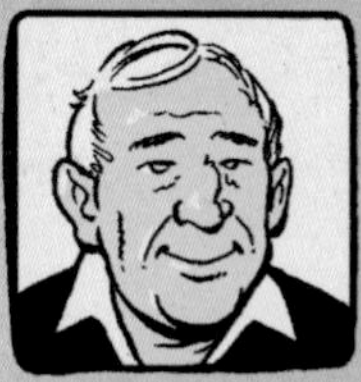

CANNABINOIDS!

TRICHOMES ALSO SYNTHESIZE COMPOUNDS THAT BIND TO RECEPTORS IN YOUR BRAIN AND THROUGHOUT YOUR BODY.

THE MOST FAMOUS OF ALL...

DR. RAPHAEL MECHOULAM

FIRST TO DISCOVER THC

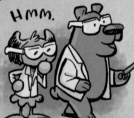

HMM.

EMPLOYEE OF THE MONTH:

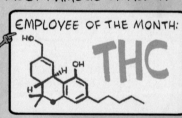

THIS CANNABINOID IS THE PRINCIPLE COMPOUND RESPONSIBLE FOR THE PSYCHOACTIVE EFFECTS OF CANNABIS

THC (TETRAHYDROCANNABINOL) & **CBD** (CANNABIDIOL) ARE ONLY **2** OF OVER **100** DIFFERENT CANNABINOIDS CURRENTLY KNOWN TO BE FOUND IN CANNABIS.

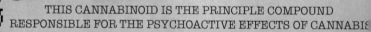

GRINDERS

FOR A NICELY ROLLED JOINT WE WANT OUR FLOWER TO BE AN EVEN CONSISTENCY, GETTING RID OF STEMS AND ANY STRAY SEEDS IN THE PROCESS.

SOME GRINDERS HAVE A CHAMBER DESIGNED TO CATCH KIEF.*
(* TRICHOMES SEPARATED FROM THE FLOWER)
KIEF CAN BE ADDED TO GROUND FLOWER FOR EXTRA POTENCY.

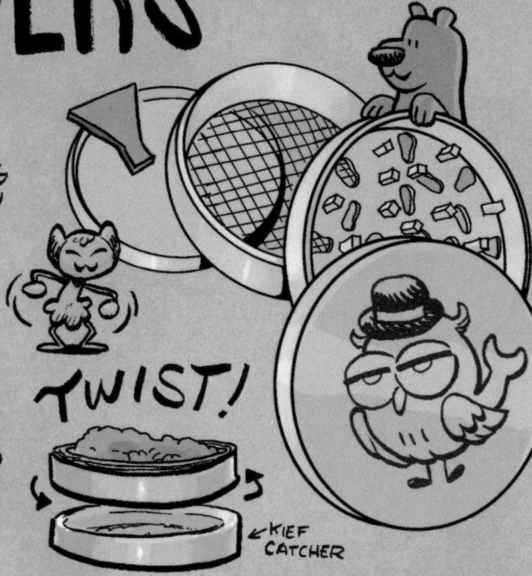
TWIST!
KIEF CATCHER

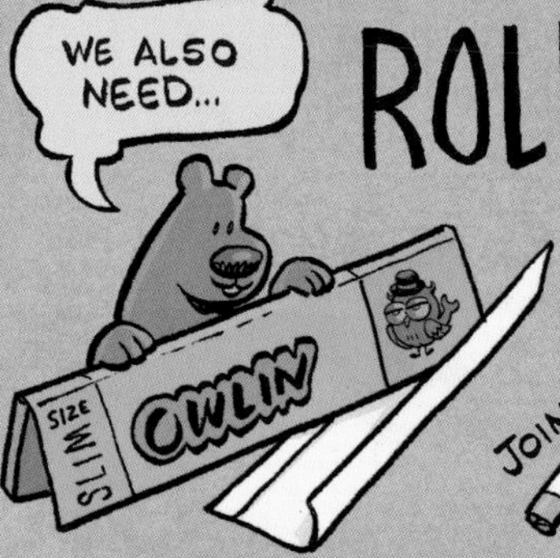
WE ALSO NEED...
SIZE
SLIM
OWLIN

ROLLING PAPERS!

THE VARIETY OF ROLLING PAPERS IS NEARLY ENDLESS—EVERYTHING FROM "BLUEBERRY-BANANA" FLAVORS TO NOVELTY SIZED "GIANT JOINT" PAPERS.

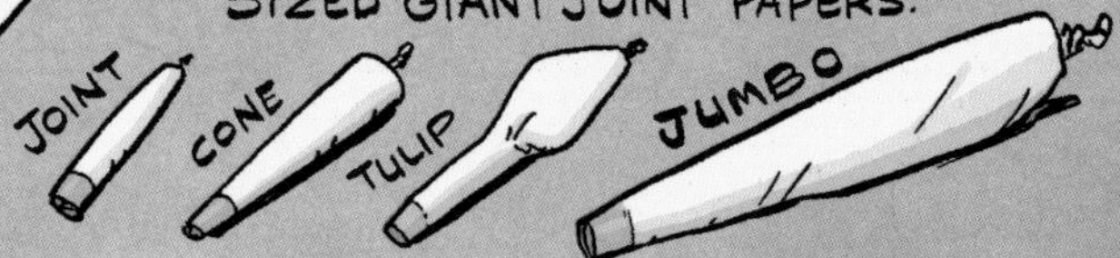
JOINT
CONE
TULIP
JUMBO

AND PAPER FILTERS

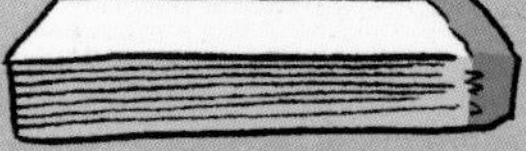

I LIKE TO USE A BASIC PAPER FILTER TO HELP KEEP TAR FROM MY LIPS.

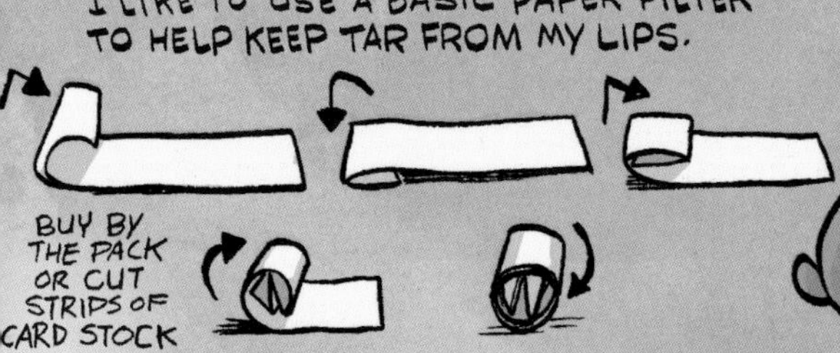

BUY BY THE PACK OR CUT STRIPS OF CARD STOCK

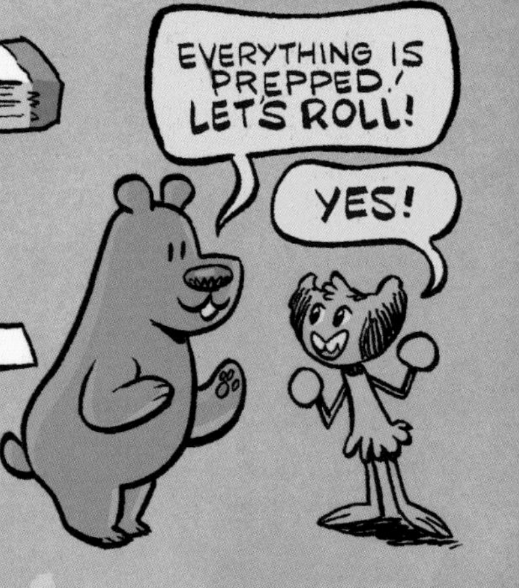
EVERYTHING IS PREPPED! LET'S ROLL!
YES!

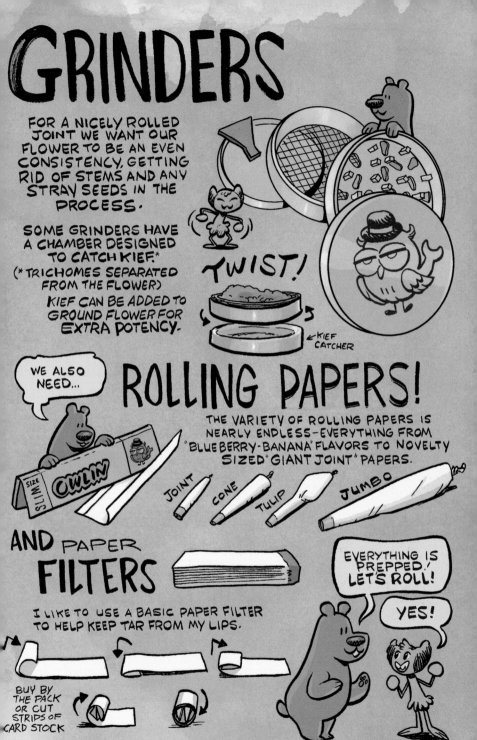

HOW TO ROLL A JOINT: BASIC EASY MODE

1. FOLD PAPER IN HALF TO CREATE A CHANNEL FOR THE FLOWER.

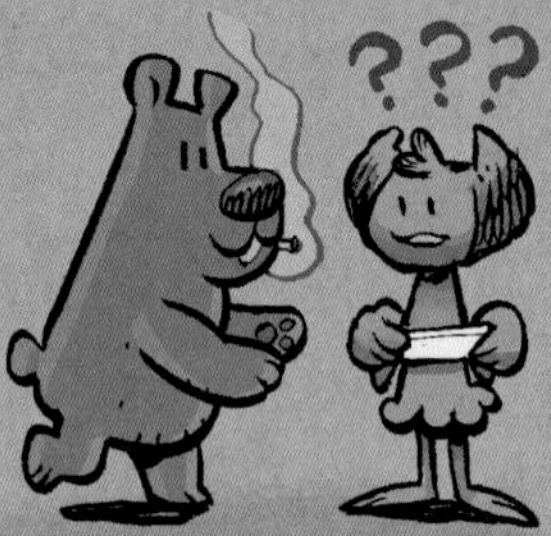
???

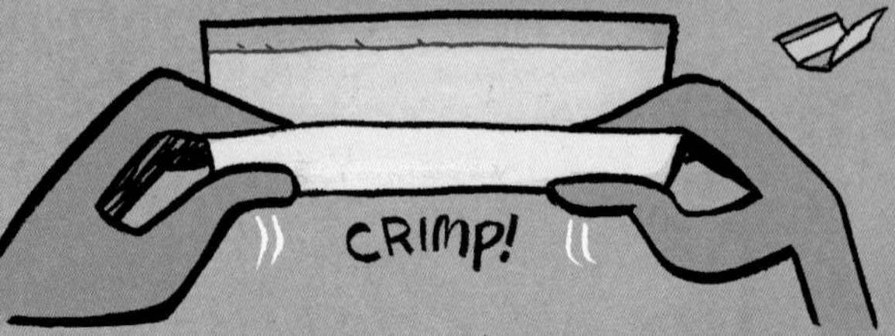
CRIMP!

ADHESIVE SIDE UP, FACING YOU.

2. USE AT LEAST HALF A GRAM, THIS DEPENDS ON THE SIZE OF YOUR PAPERS, REALLY.

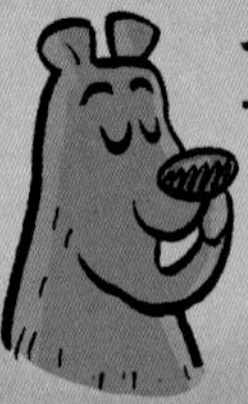

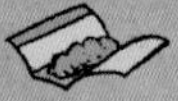

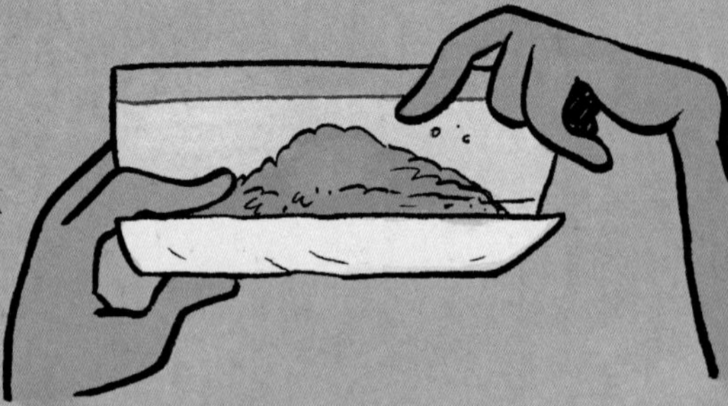

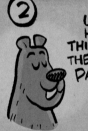

LEAVE ROOM ON THE ENDS FOR YOUR FILTER AND "HAT."

3. HOLD EACH END WITH YOUR FINGERS, ROCKING GENTLY TO EVENLY DISTRIBUTE THE FLOWER AND SOFTEN THE PAPER.

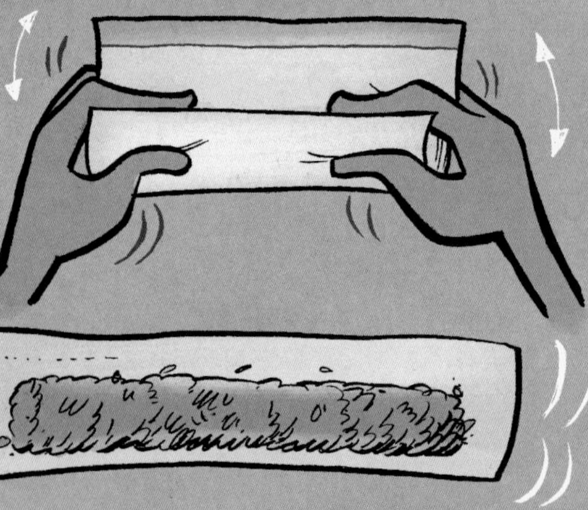

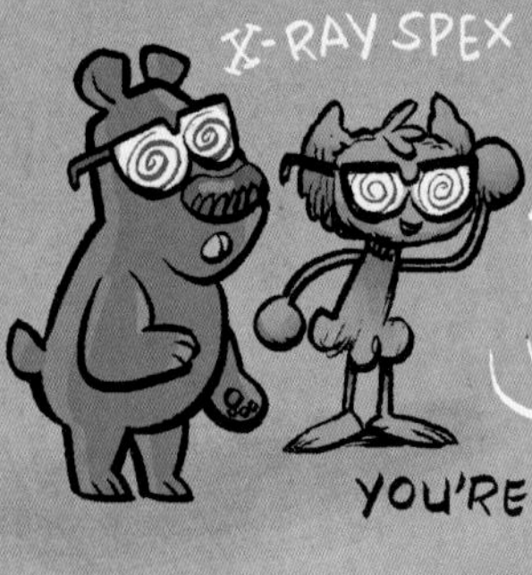
X-RAY SPEX

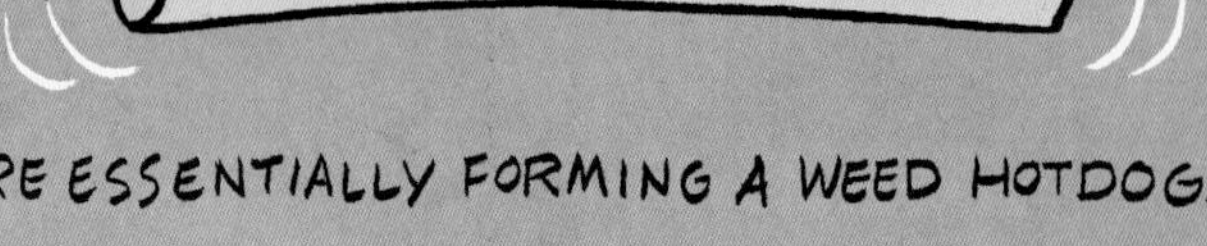

YOU'RE ESSENTIALLY FORMING A WEED HOTDOG.

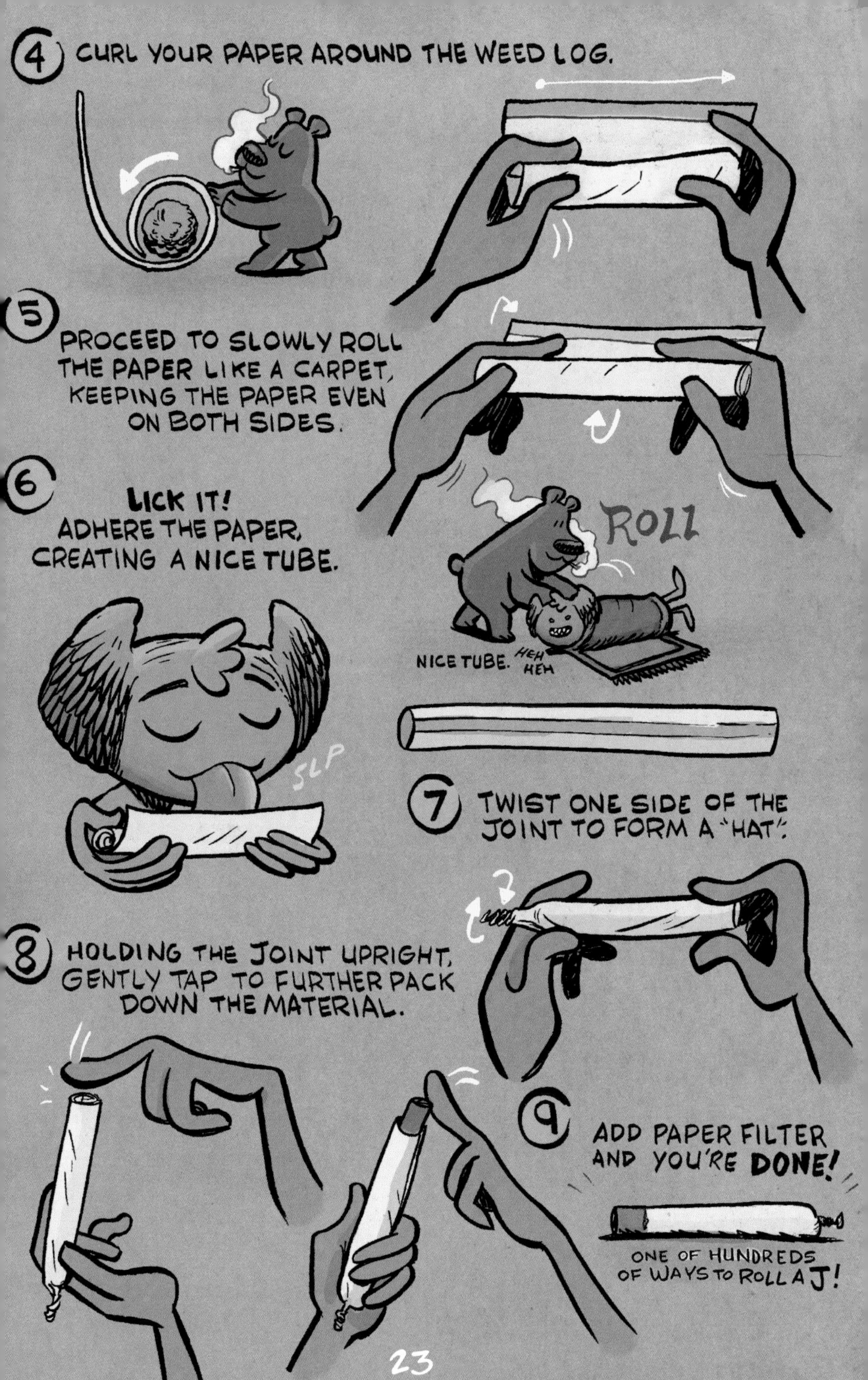
4 CURL YOUR PAPER AROUND THE WEED LOG.
5 PROCEED TO SLOWLY ROLL THE PAPER LIKE A CARPET, KEEPING THE PAPER EVEN ON BOTH SIDES.
6 LICK IT! ADHERE THE PAPER, CREATING A NICE TUBE.
ROLL
NICE TUBE.
HEH HEH
SLP
7 TWIST ONE SIDE OF THE JOINT TO FORM A "HAT".
8 HOLDING THE JOINT UPRIGHT, GENTLY TAP TO FURTHER PACK DOWN THE MATERIAL.
9 ADD PAPER FILTER AND YOU'RE DONE!
ONE OF HUNDREDS OF WAYS TO ROLL A J!

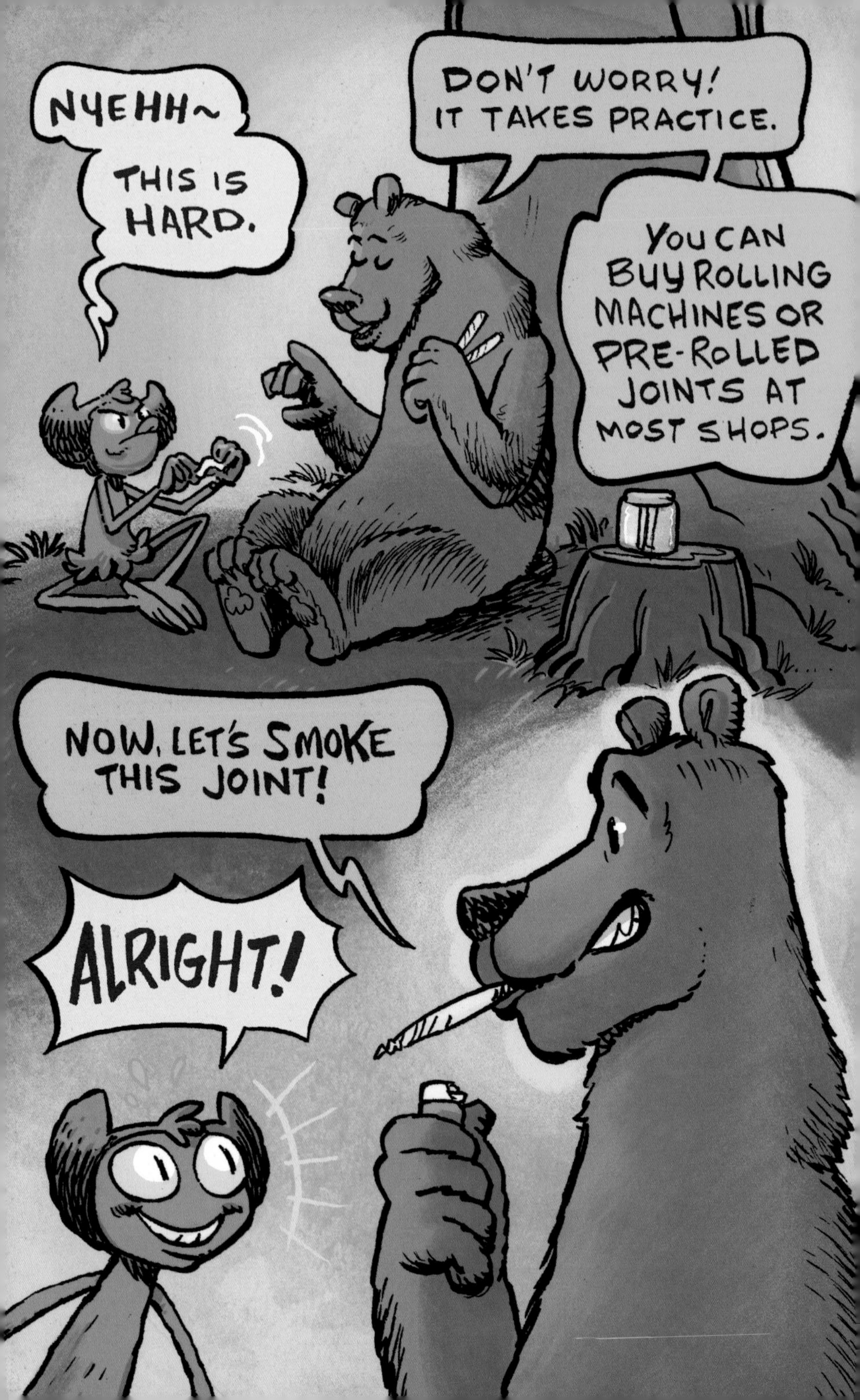
NYEHH~
THIS IS HARD.
DON'T WORRY! IT TAKES PRACTICE.
YOU CAN BUY ROLLING MACHINES OR PRE-ROLLED JOINTS AT MOST SHOPS.
NOW, LET'S SMOKE THIS JOINT!
ALRIGHT!

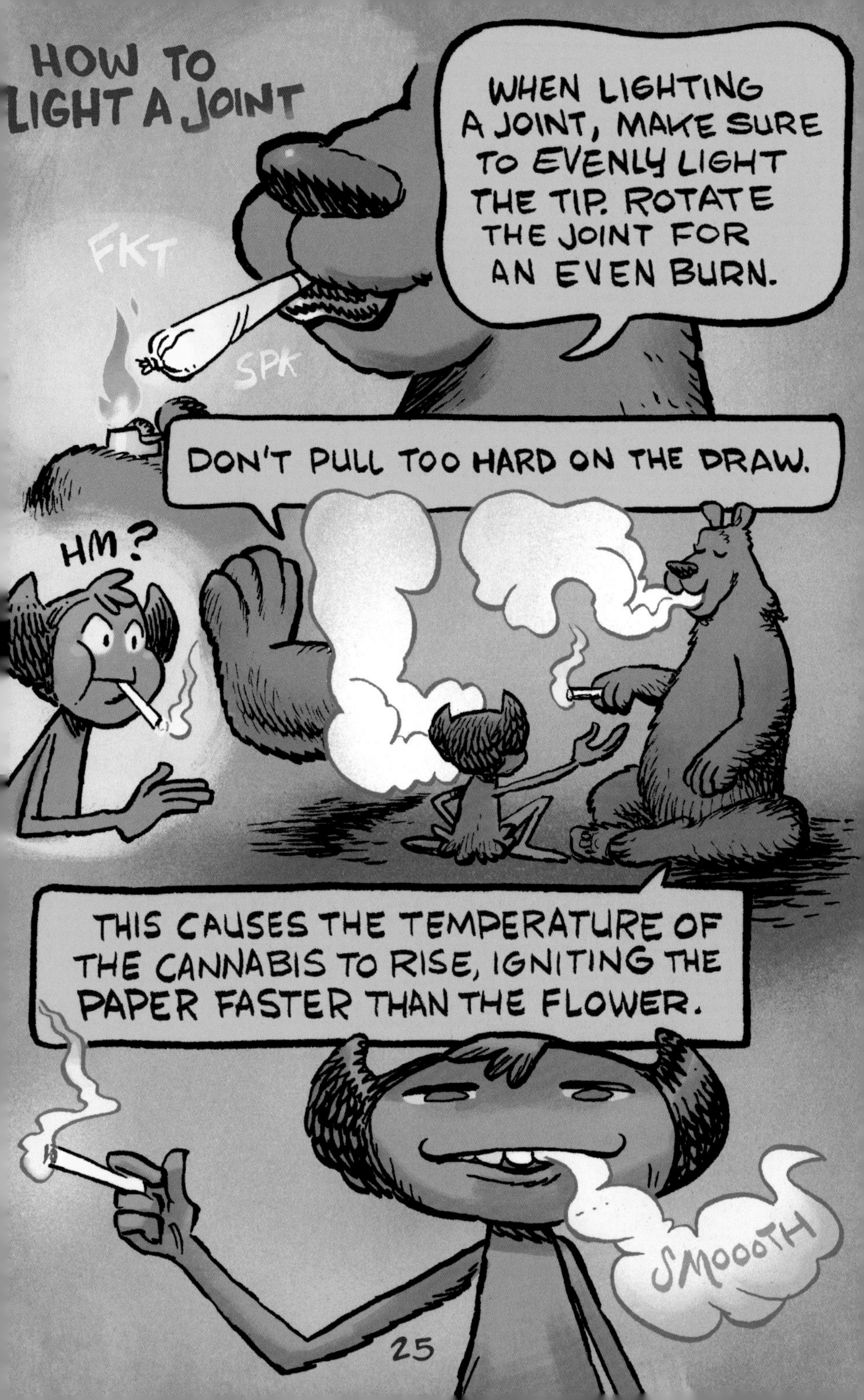
HOW TO LIGHT A JOINT
WHEN LIGHTING A JOINT, MAKE SURE TO EVENLY LIGHT THE TIP. ROTATE THE JOINT FOR AN EVEN BURN.
FKT
SPK
DON'T PULL TOO HARD ON THE DRAW.
HM?
THIS CAUSES THE TEMPERATURE OF THE CANNABIS TO RISE, IGNITING THE PAPER FASTER THAN THE FLOWER.
SMOOOTH

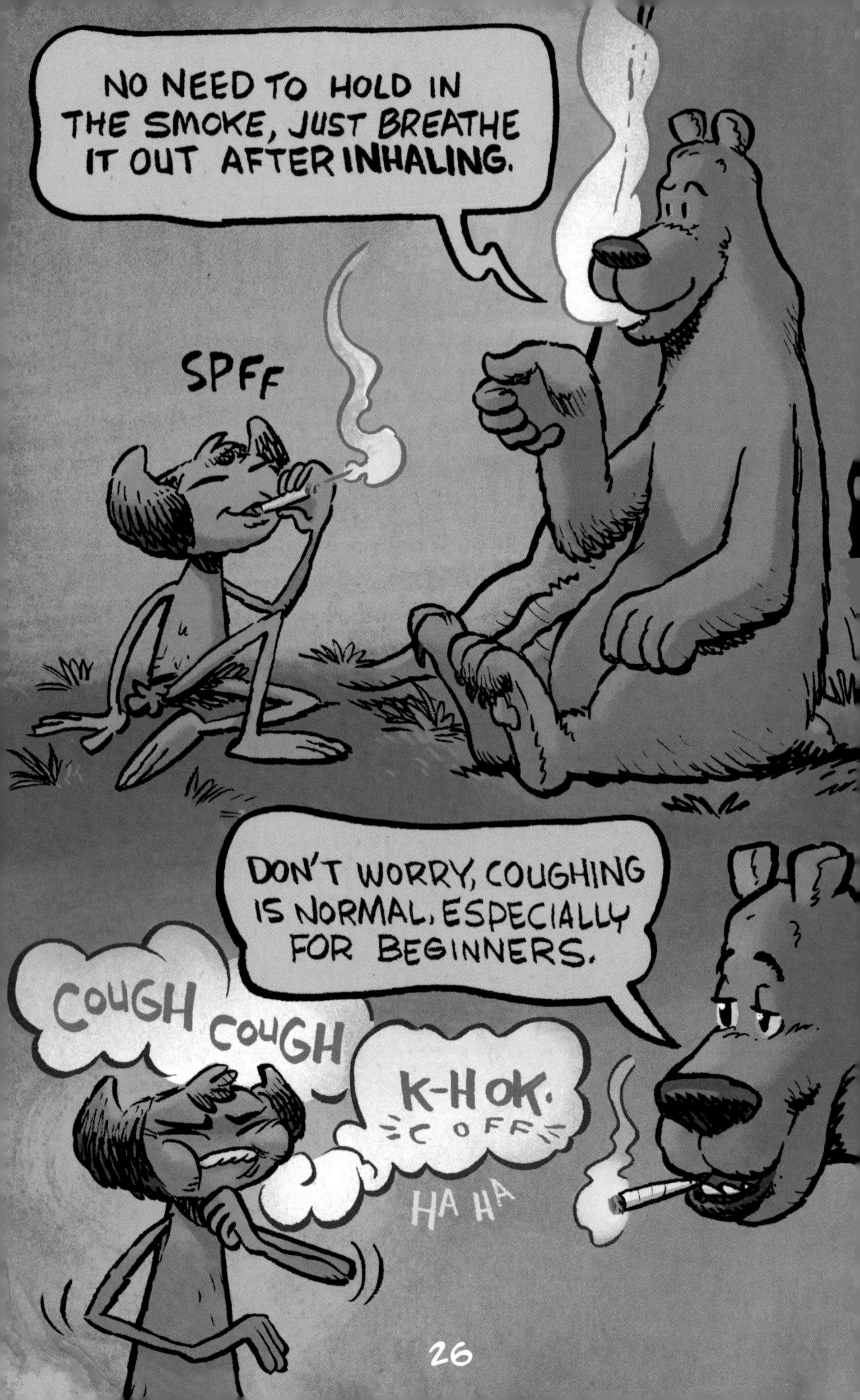
NO NEED TO HOLD IN THE SMOKE, JUST BREATHE IT OUT AFTER INHALING.
SPFF
DON'T WORRY, COUGHING IS NORMAL, ESPECIALLY FOR BEGINNERS.
COUGH COUGH
K-HOK.
COFF
HA HA

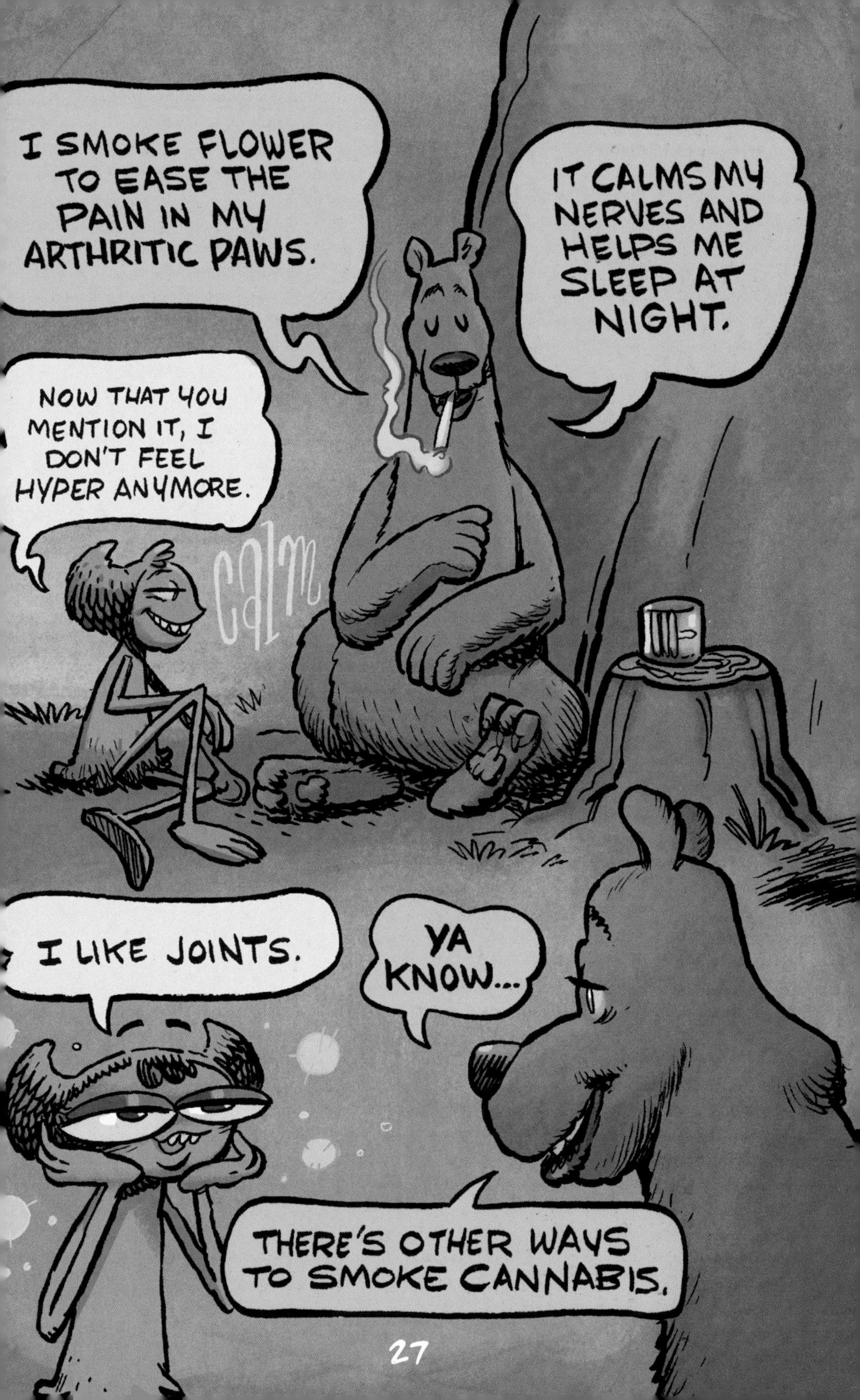
I SMOKE FLOWER TO EASE THE PAIN IN MY ARTHRITIC PAWS.
IT CALMS MY NERVES AND HELPS ME SLEEP AT NIGHT.
NOW THAT YOU MENTION IT, I DON'T FEEL HYPER ANYMORE.
calm
I LIKE JOINTS.
YA KNOW...
THERE'S OTHER WAYS TO SMOKE CANNABIS.

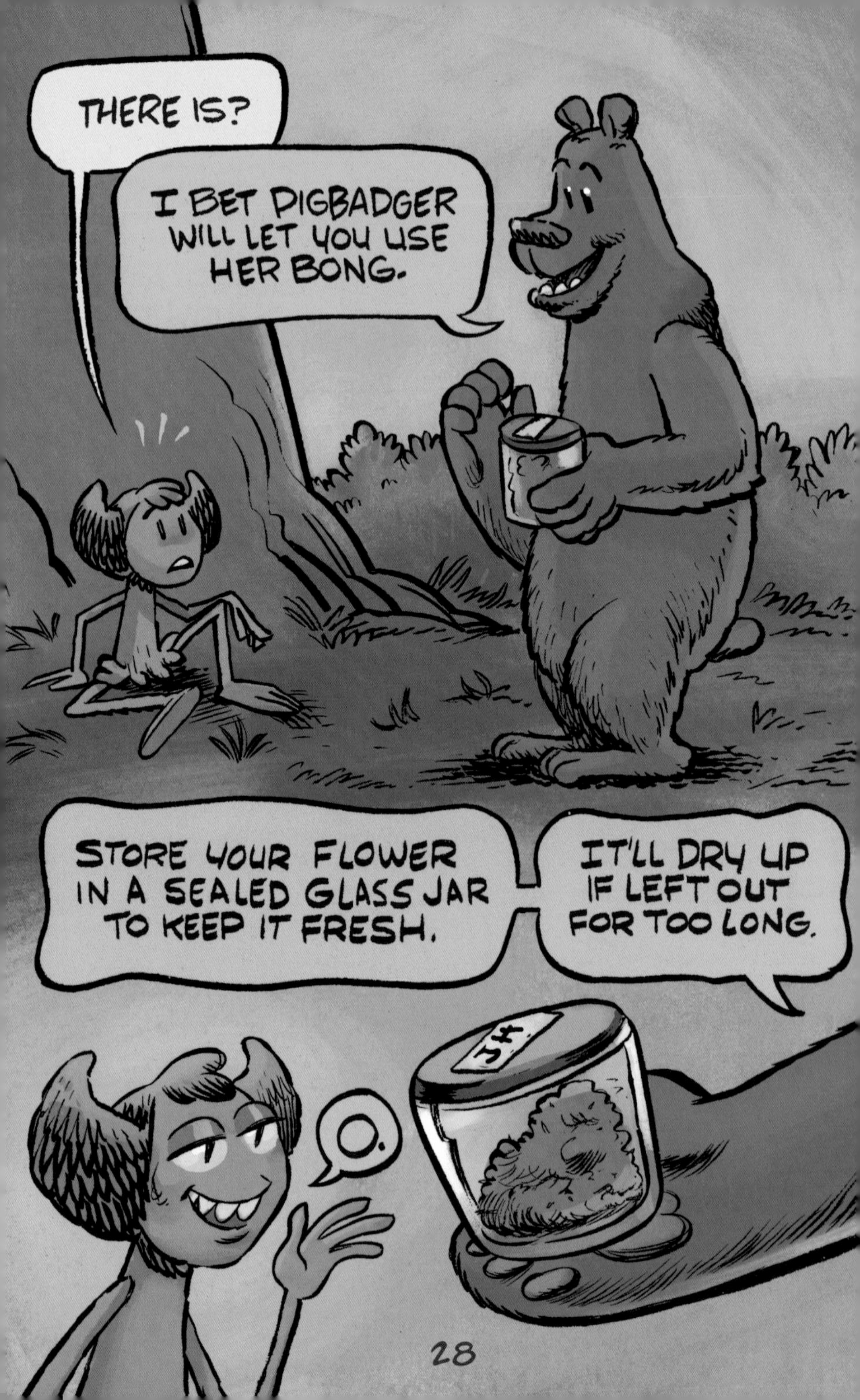
THERE IS?
I BET PIGBADGER WILL LET YOU USE HER BONG.
STORE YOUR FLOWER IN A SEALED GLASS JAR TO KEEP IT FRESH.
IT'LL DRY UP IF LEFT OUT FOR TOO LONG.
O.

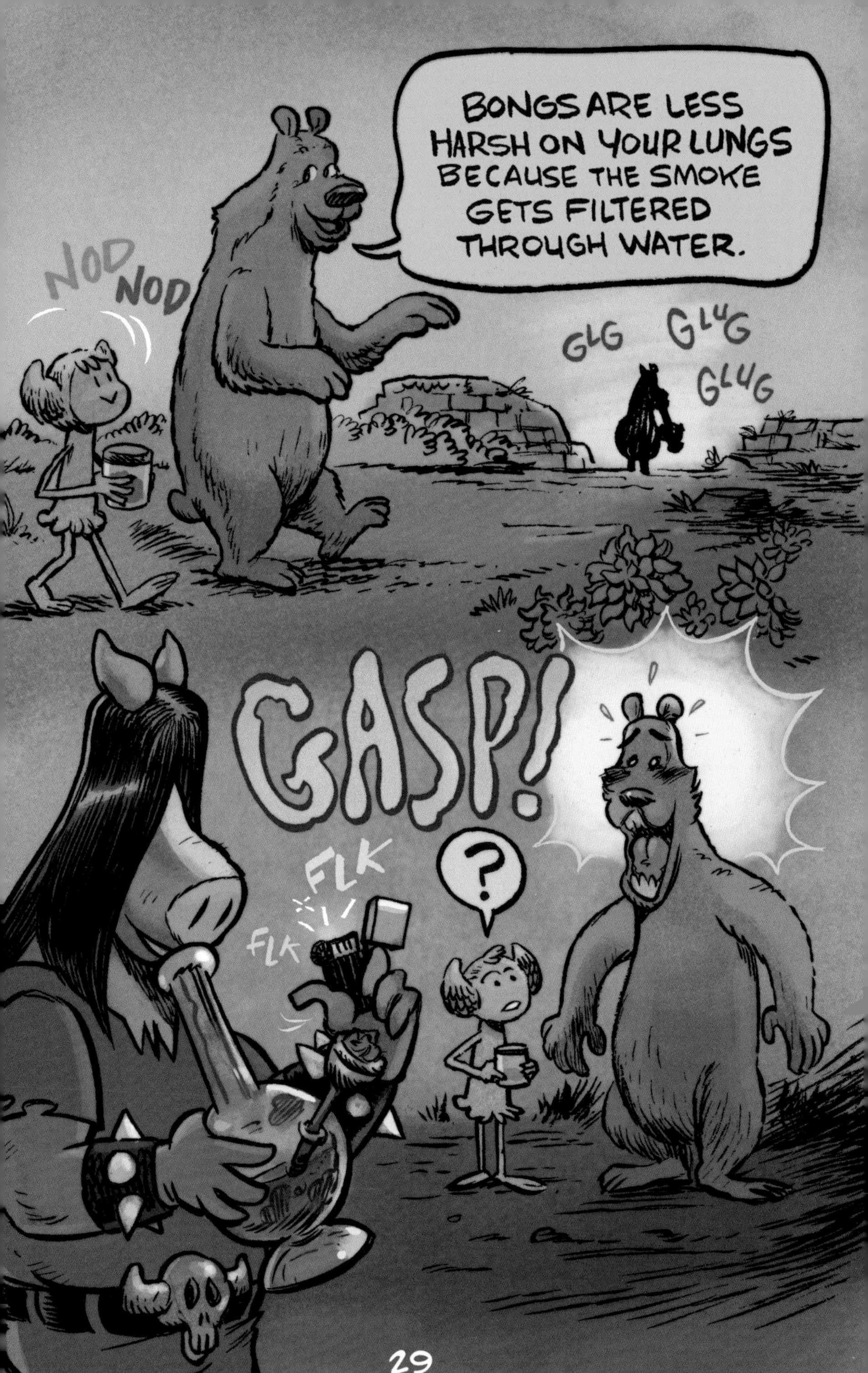
BONGS ARE LESS HARSH ON YOUR LUNGS BECAUSE THE SMOKE GETS FILTERED THROUGH WATER.
NOD NOD
GLG GLUG GLUG
GASP!
FLK
FLK
?

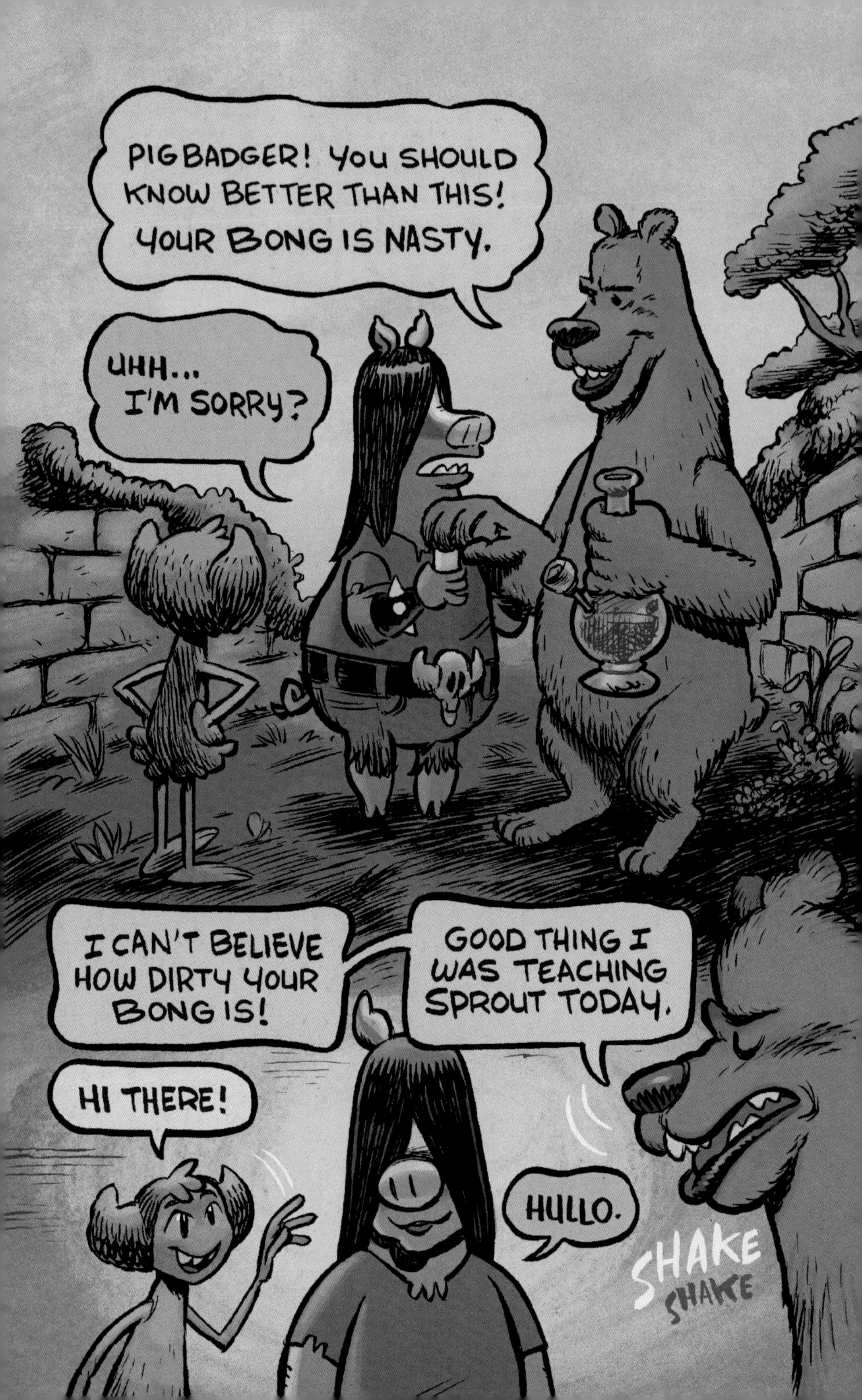
PIGBADGER! YOU SHOULD KNOW BETTER THAN THIS! YOUR BONG IS NASTY.
UHH... I'M SORRY?
I CAN'T BELIEVE HOW DIRTY YOUR BONG IS!
GOOD THING I WAS TEACHING SPROUT TODAY.
HI THERE!
HULLO.
SHAKE
SHAKE

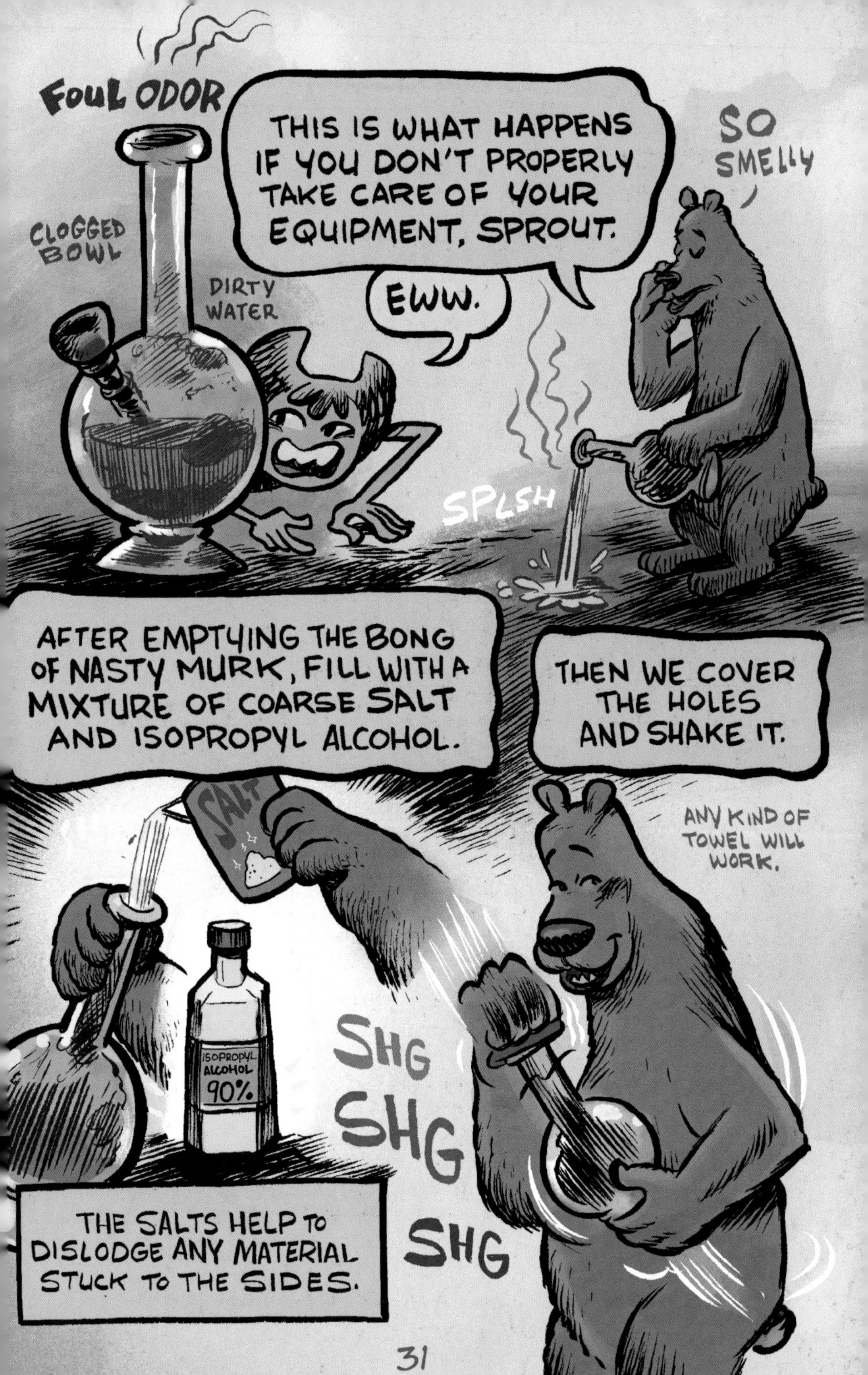
FOUL ODOR
CLOGGED BOWL
DIRTY WATER
THIS IS WHAT HAPPENS IF YOU DON'T PROPERLY TAKE CARE OF YOUR EQUIPMENT, SPROUT.
EWW.
SO SMELLY
SPLSH
AFTER EMPTYING THE BONG OF NASTY MURK, FILL WITH A MIXTURE OF COARSE SALT AND ISOPROPYL ALCOHOL.
THEN WE COVER THE HOLES AND SHAKE IT.
SALT
ANY KIND OF TOWEL WILL WORK.
ISOPROPYL ALCOHOL 90%
SHG
SHG
SHG
THE SALTS HELP TO DISLODGE ANY MATERIAL STUCK TO THE SIDES.

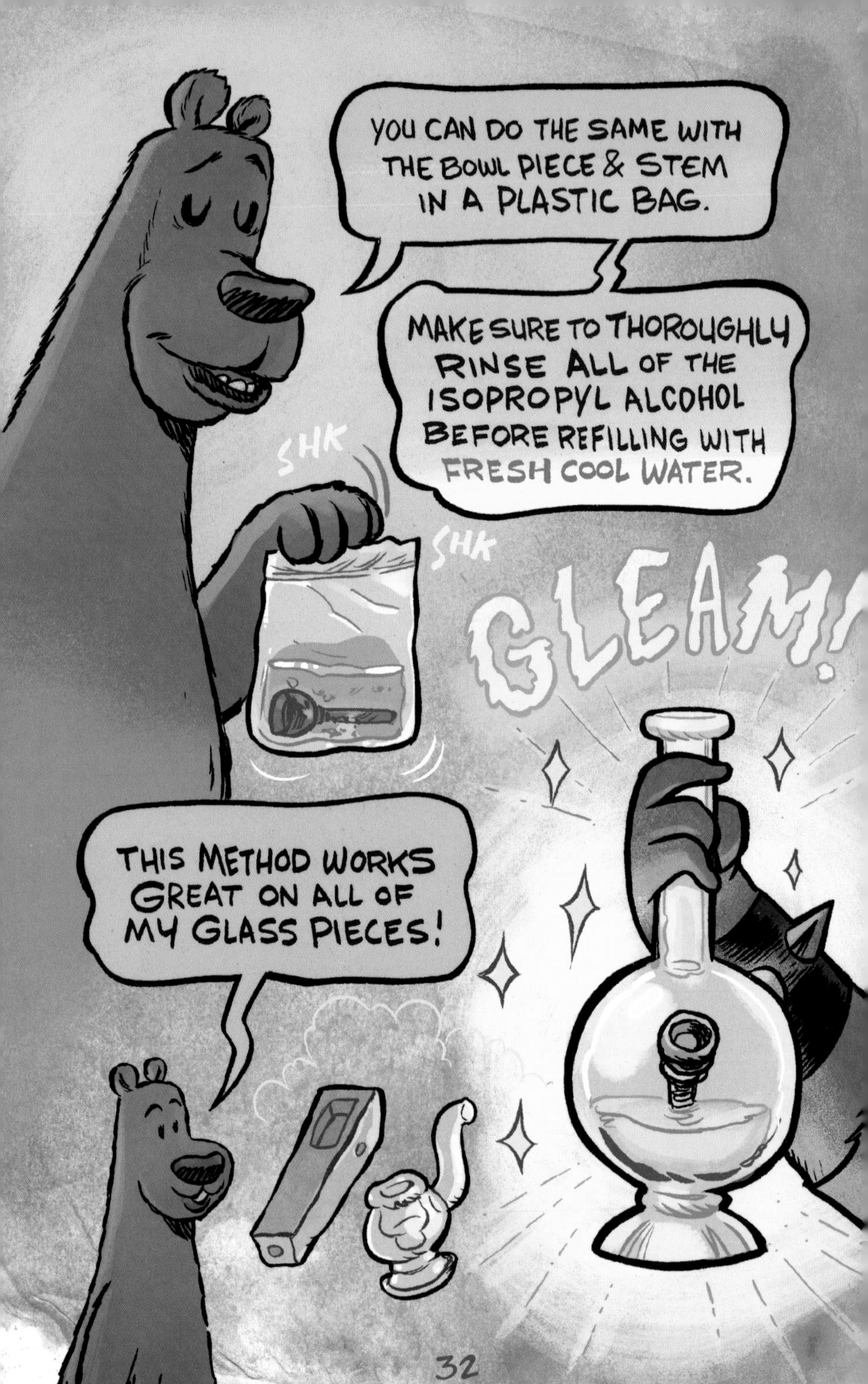
YOU CAN DO THE SAME WITH THE BOWL PIECE & STEM IN A PLASTIC BAG.
MAKE SURE TO THOROUGHLY RINSE ALL OF THE ISOPROPYL ALCOHOL BEFORE REFILLING WITH FRESH COOL WATER.
SHK
SHK
GLEAM!
THIS METHOD WORKS GREAT ON ALL OF MY GLASS PIECES!

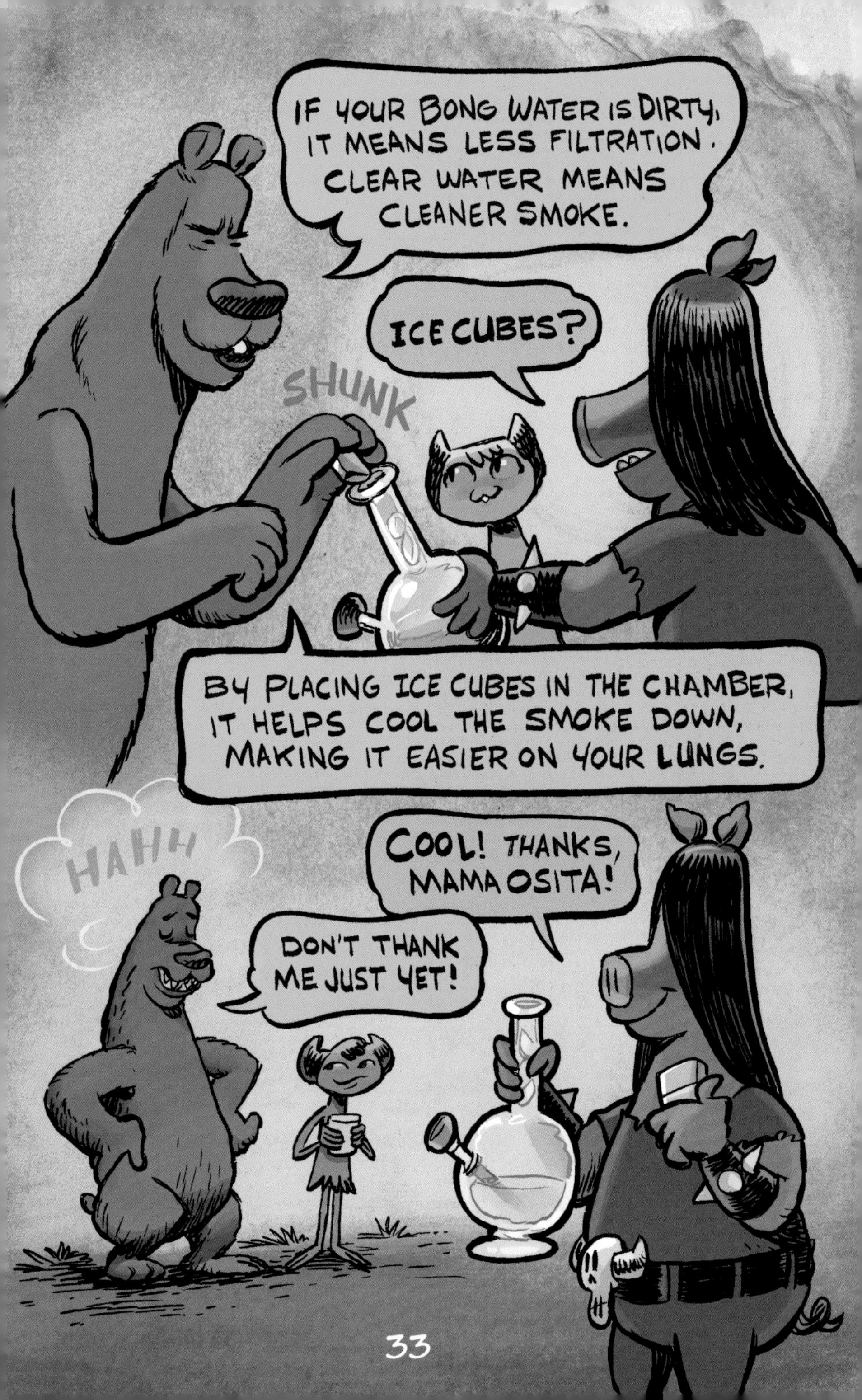
IF YOUR BONG WATER IS DIRTY, IT MEANS LESS FILTRATION. CLEAR WATER MEANS CLEANER SMOKE.
ICE CUBES?
SHUNK
BY PLACING ICE CUBES IN THE CHAMBER, IT HELPS COOL THE SMOKE DOWN, MAKING IT EASIER ON YOUR LUNGS.
HAHH
COOL! THANKS, MAMA OSITA!
DON'T THANK ME JUST YET!

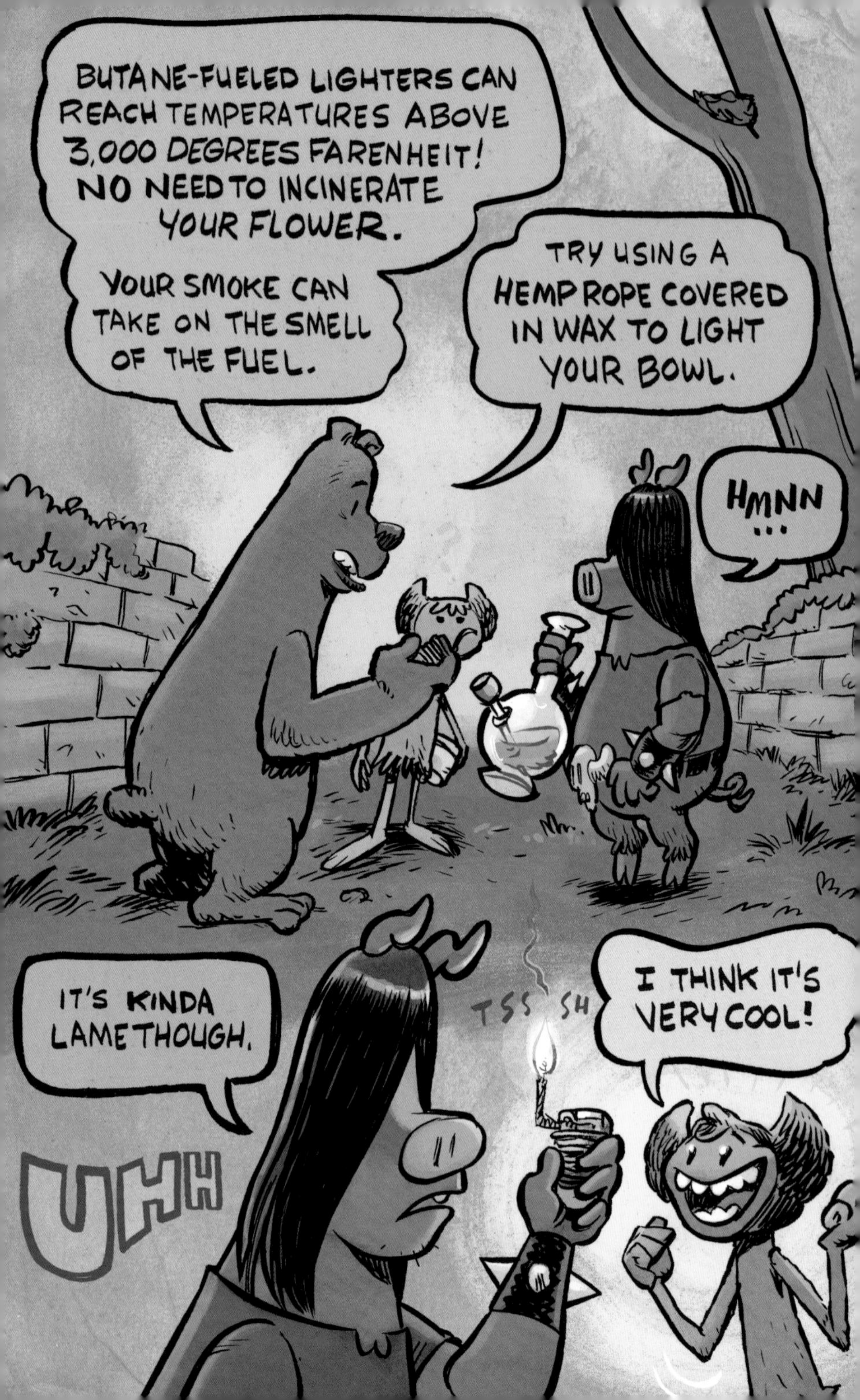
BUTANE-FUELED LIGHTERS CAN REACH TEMPERATURES ABOVE 3,000 DEGREES FARENHEIT! NO NEED TO INCINERATE YOUR FLOWER.
YOUR SMOKE CAN TAKE ON THE SMELL OF THE FUEL.
TRY USING A HEMP ROPE COVERED IN WAX TO LIGHT YOUR BOWL.
HMNN...
IT'S KINDA LAME THOUGH.
UHH
TSSSH
I THINK IT'S VERY COOL!

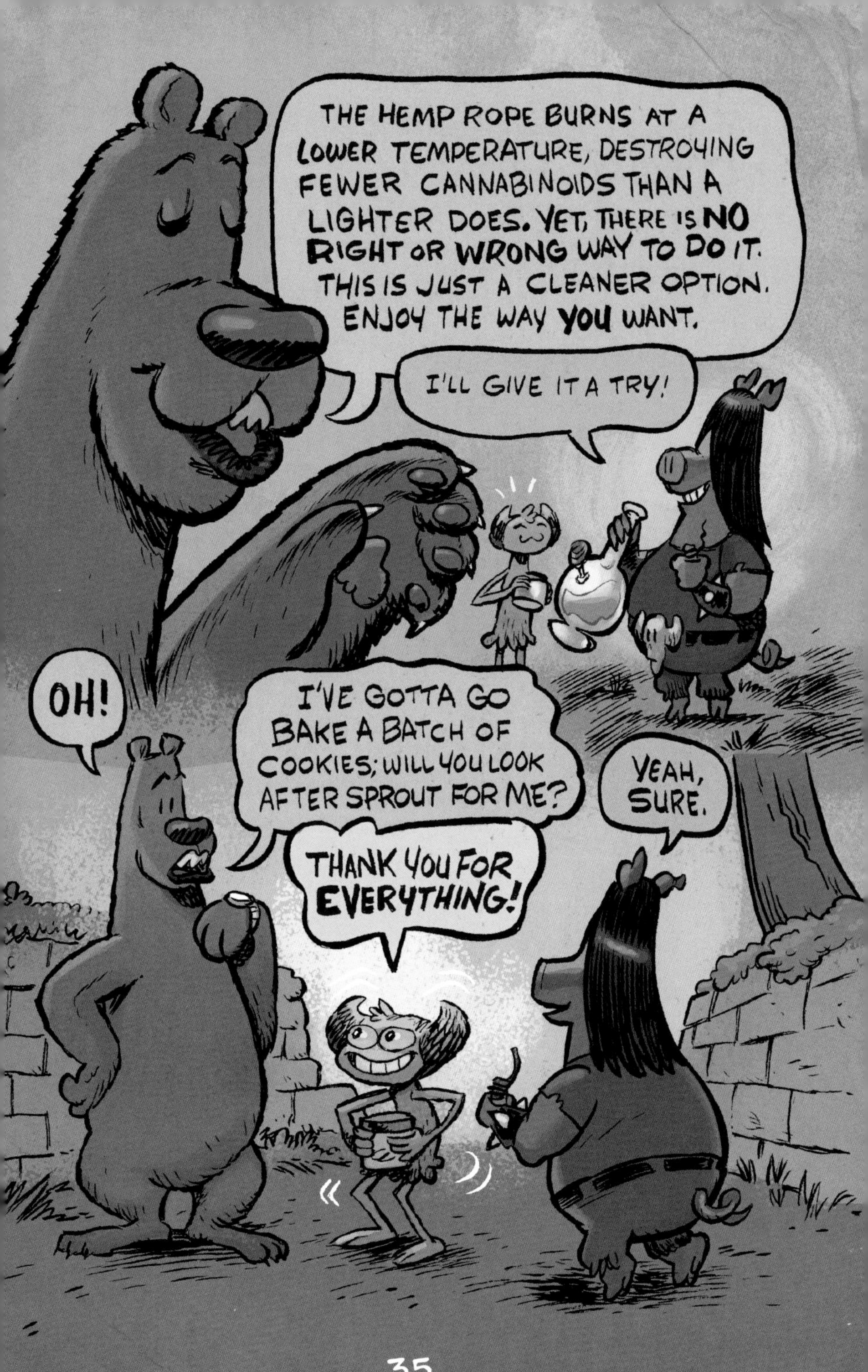
THE HEMP ROPE BURNS AT A LOWER TEMPERATURE, DESTROYING FEWER CANNABINOIDS THAN A LIGHTER DOES. YET, THERE IS NO RIGHT OR WRONG WAY TO DO IT. THIS IS JUST A CLEANER OPTION. ENJOY THE WAY YOU WANT.
I'LL GIVE IT A TRY!
OH!
I'VE GOTTA GO BAKE A BATCH OF COOKIES; WILL YOU LOOK AFTER SPROUT FOR ME?
YEAH, SURE.
THANK YOU FOR EVERYTHING!

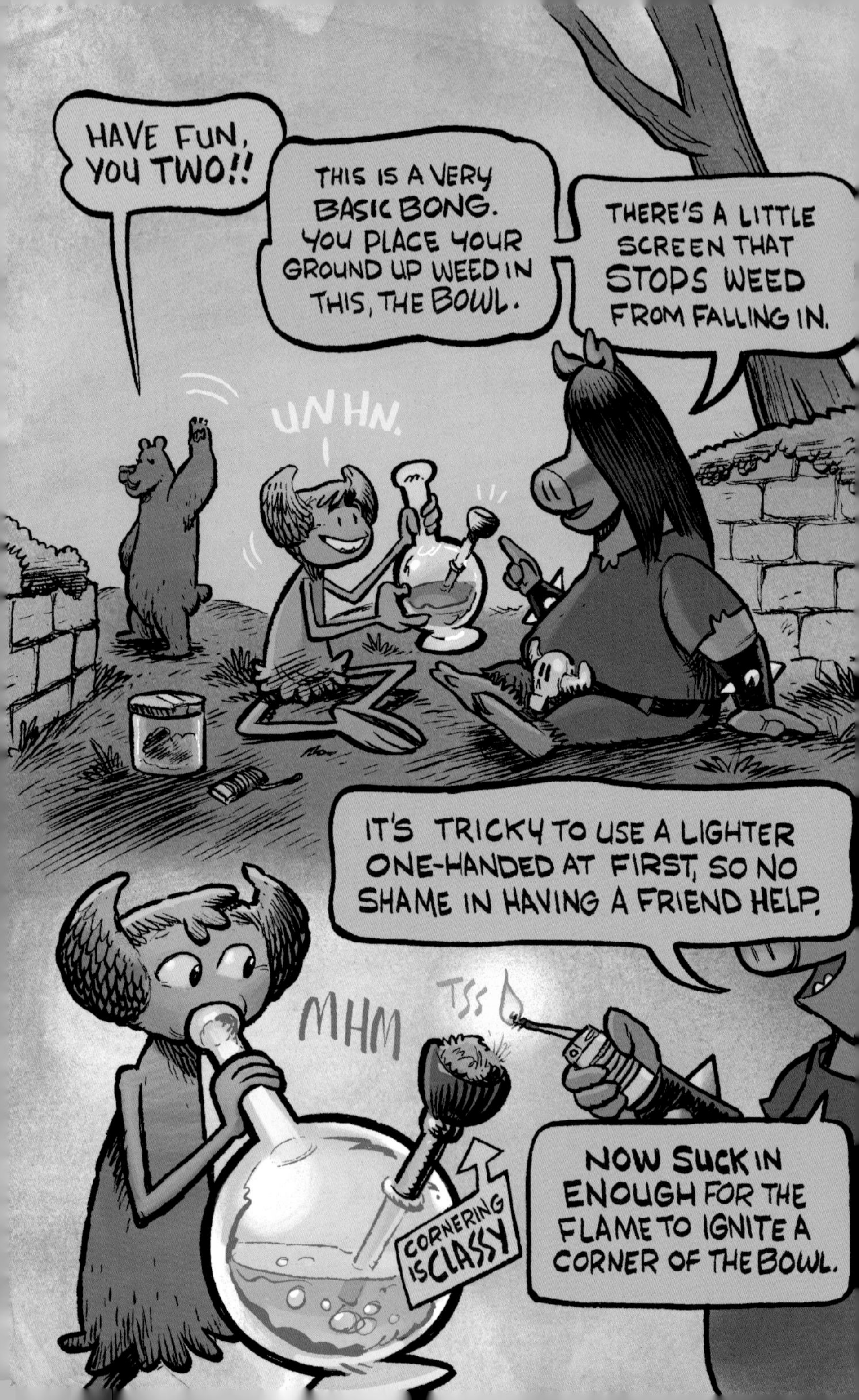
HAVE FUN, YOU TWO!!
THIS IS A VERY BASIC BONG. YOU PLACE YOUR GROUND UP WEED IN THIS, THE BOWL.
THERE'S A LITTLE SCREEN THAT STOPS WEED FROM FALLING IN.
UNHN.
IT'S TRICKY TO USE A LIGHTER ONE-HANDED AT FIRST, SO NO SHAME IN HAVING A FRIEND HELP.
MHM
TSS
CORNERING IS CLASSY
NOW SUCK IN ENOUGH FOR THE FLAME TO IGNITE A CORNER OF THE BOWL.

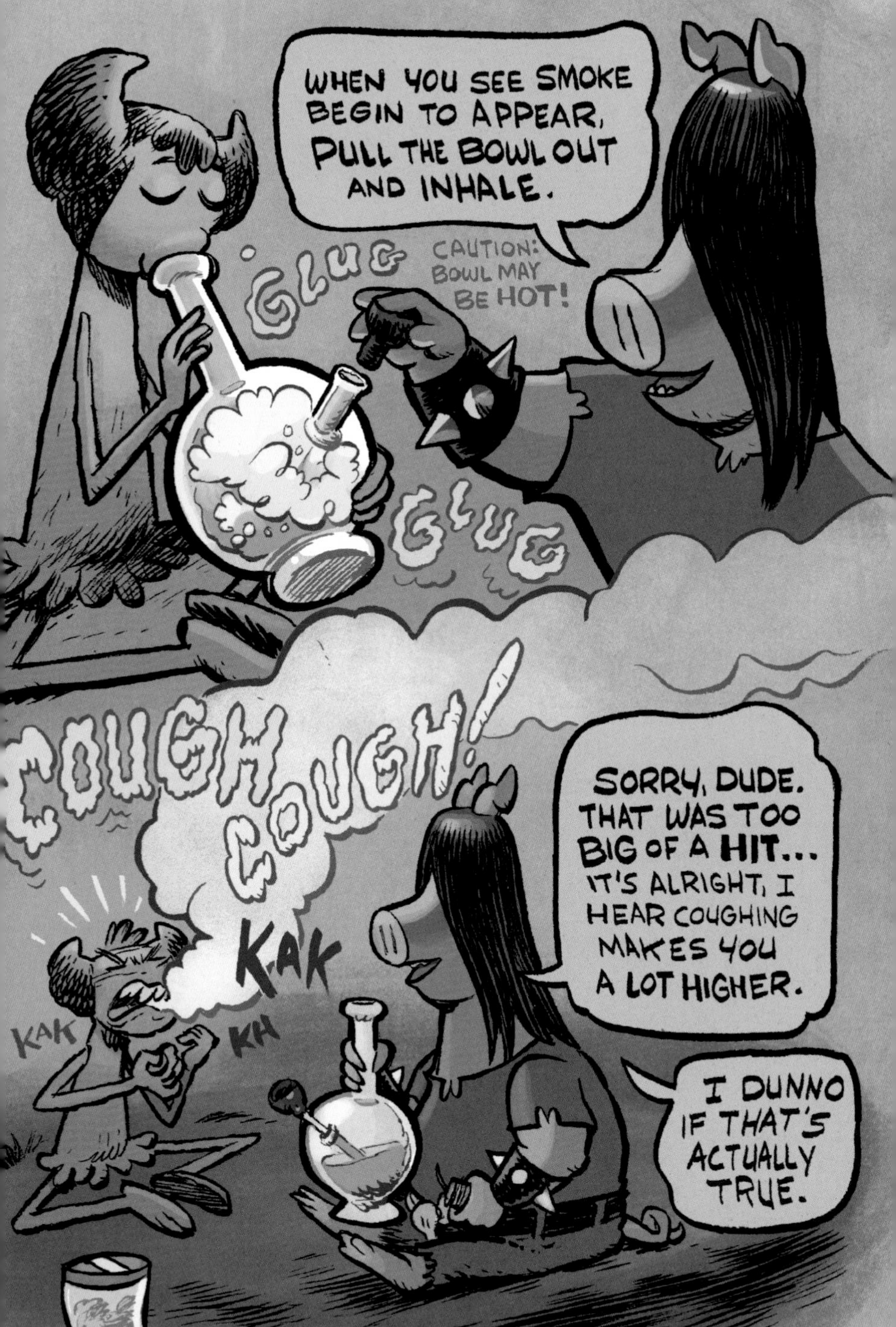
WHEN YOU SEE SMOKE BEGIN TO APPEAR, PULL THE BOWL OUT AND INHALE.
GLUG
CAUTION: BOWL MAY BE HOT!
GLUG
COUGH COUGH!
KAK
KAK
KH
SORRY, DUDE. THAT WAS TOO BIG OF A HIT...
IT'S ALRIGHT, I HEAR COUGHING MAKES YOU A LOT HIGHER.
I DUNNO IF THAT'S ACTUALLY TRUE.

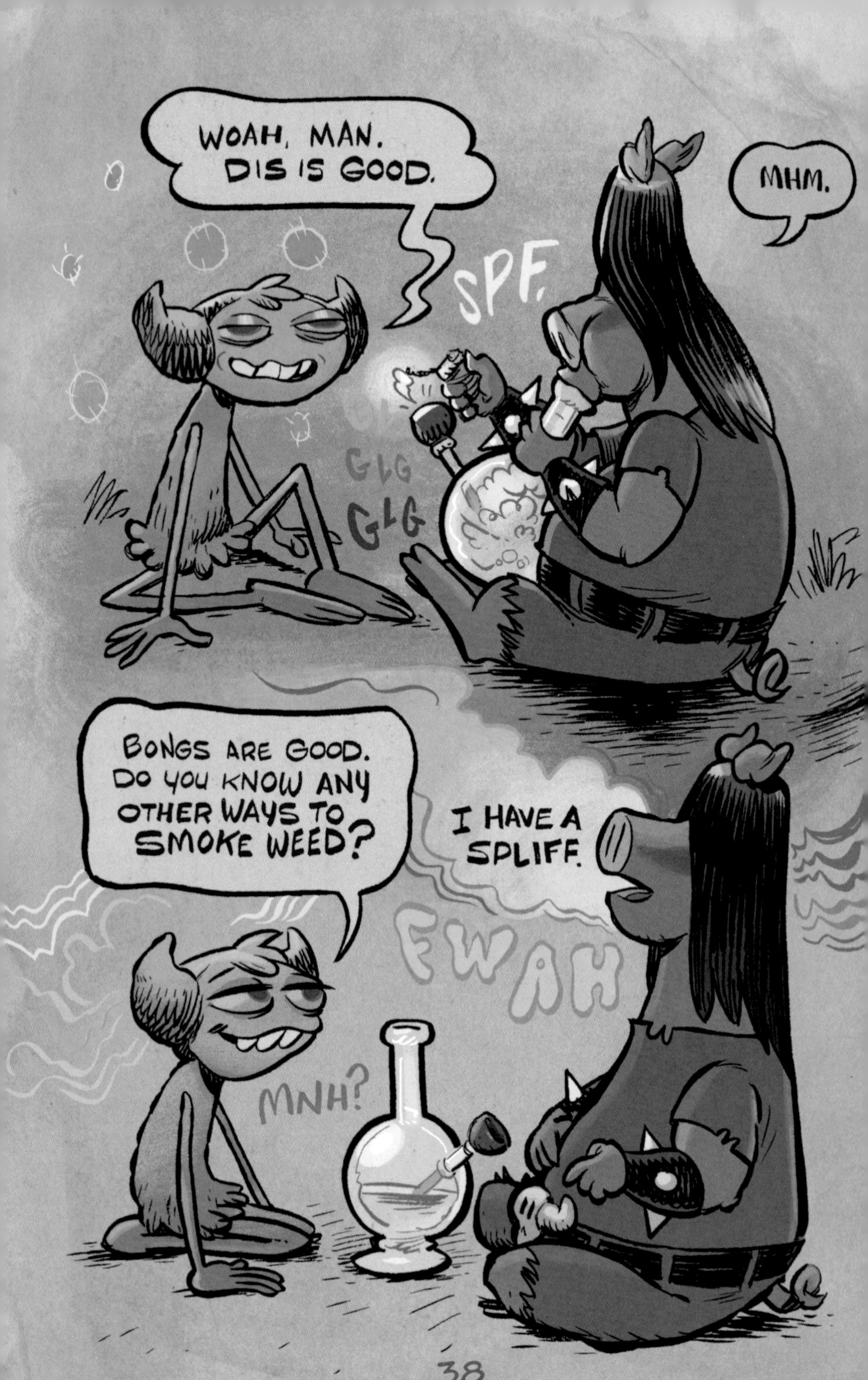
WOAH, MAN. DIS IS GOOD.
MHM.
SPF.
GLG
GLG
BONGS ARE GOOD. DO YOU KNOW ANY OTHER WAYS TO SMOKE WEED?
I HAVE A SPLIFF.
FWAH
MNH?

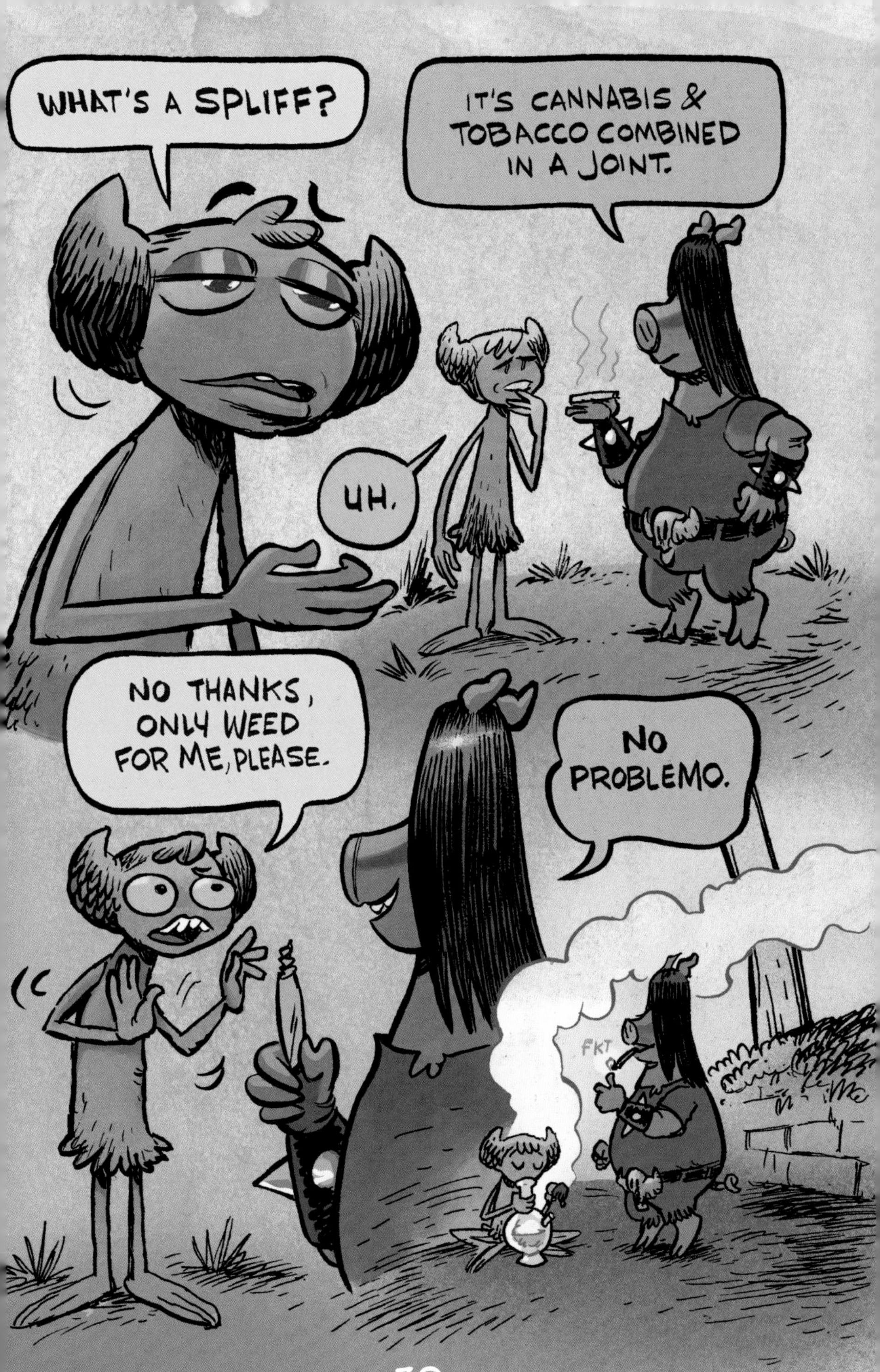
WHAT'S A SPLIFF?
IT'S CANNABIS & TOBACCO COMBINED IN A JOINT.
UH.
NO THANKS, ONLY WEED FOR ME, PLEASE.
NO PROBLEMO.
FKT

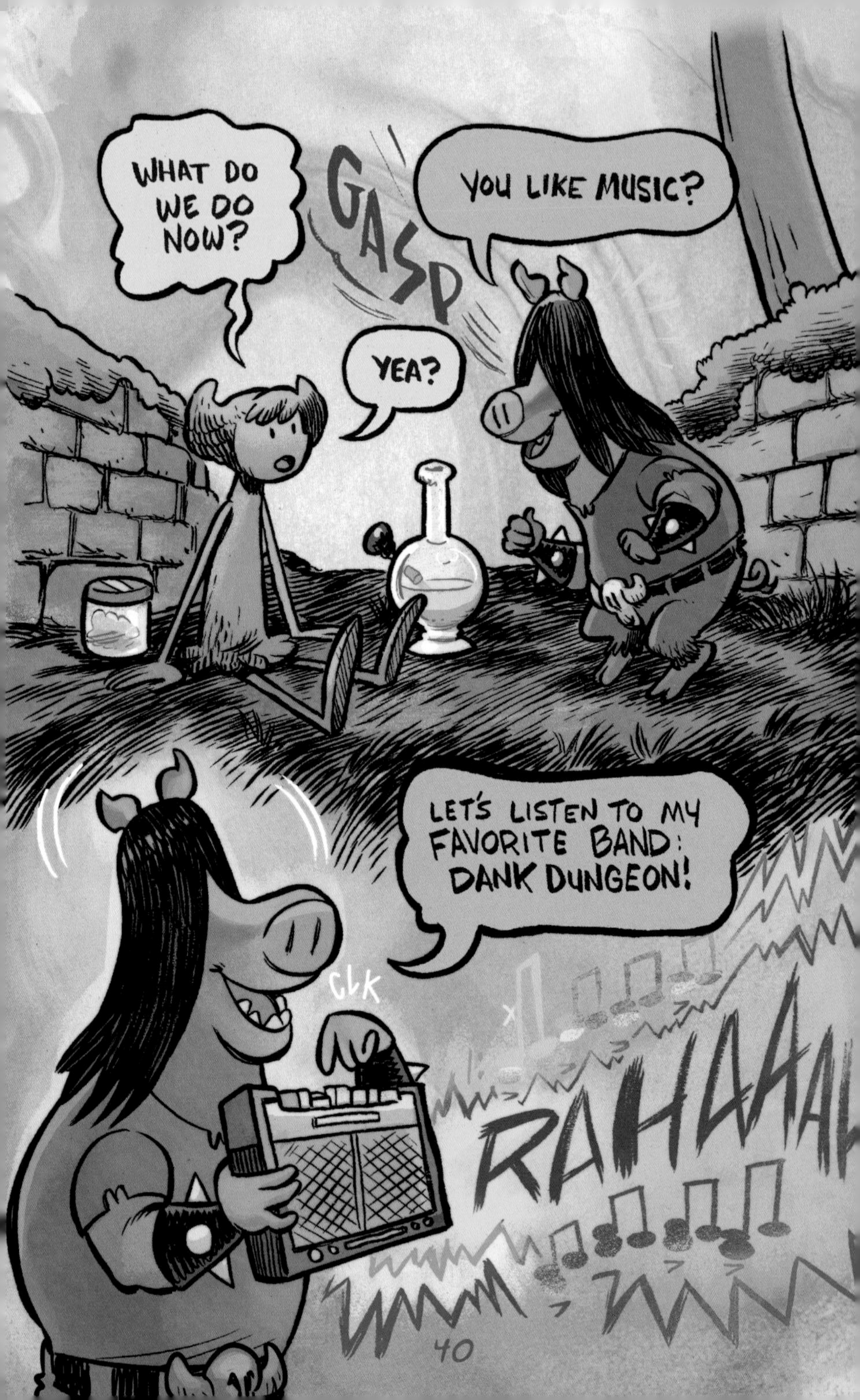
WHAT DO WE DO NOW?
GASP
YOU LIKE MUSIC?
YEA?
LET'S LISTEN TO MY FAVORITE BAND: DANK DUNGEON!
CLK
RAHAA

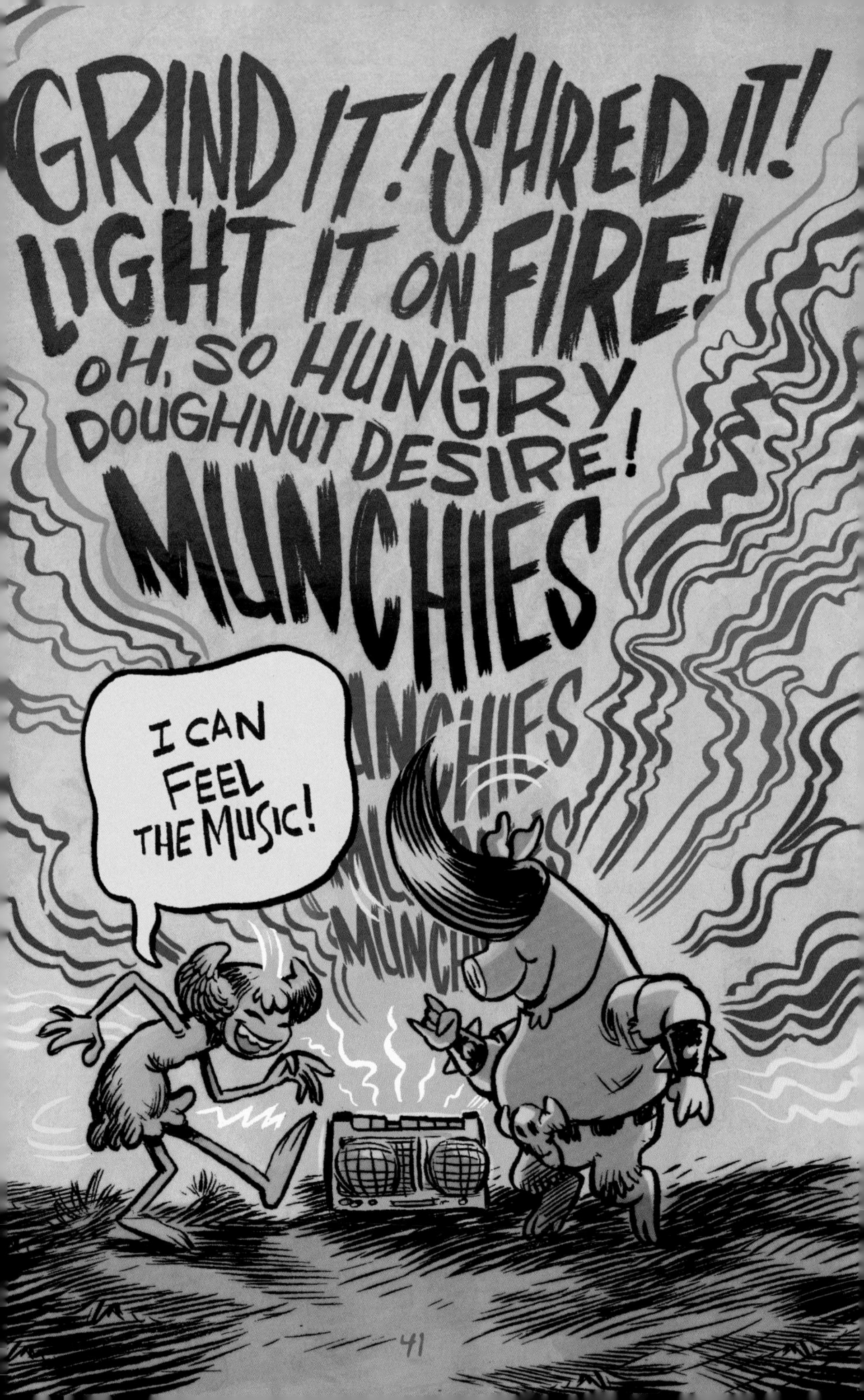
GRIND IT! SHRED IT!
LIGHT IT ON FIRE!
OH, SO HUNGRY
DOUGHNUT DESIRE!
MUNCHIES
I CAN FEEL THE MUSIC!

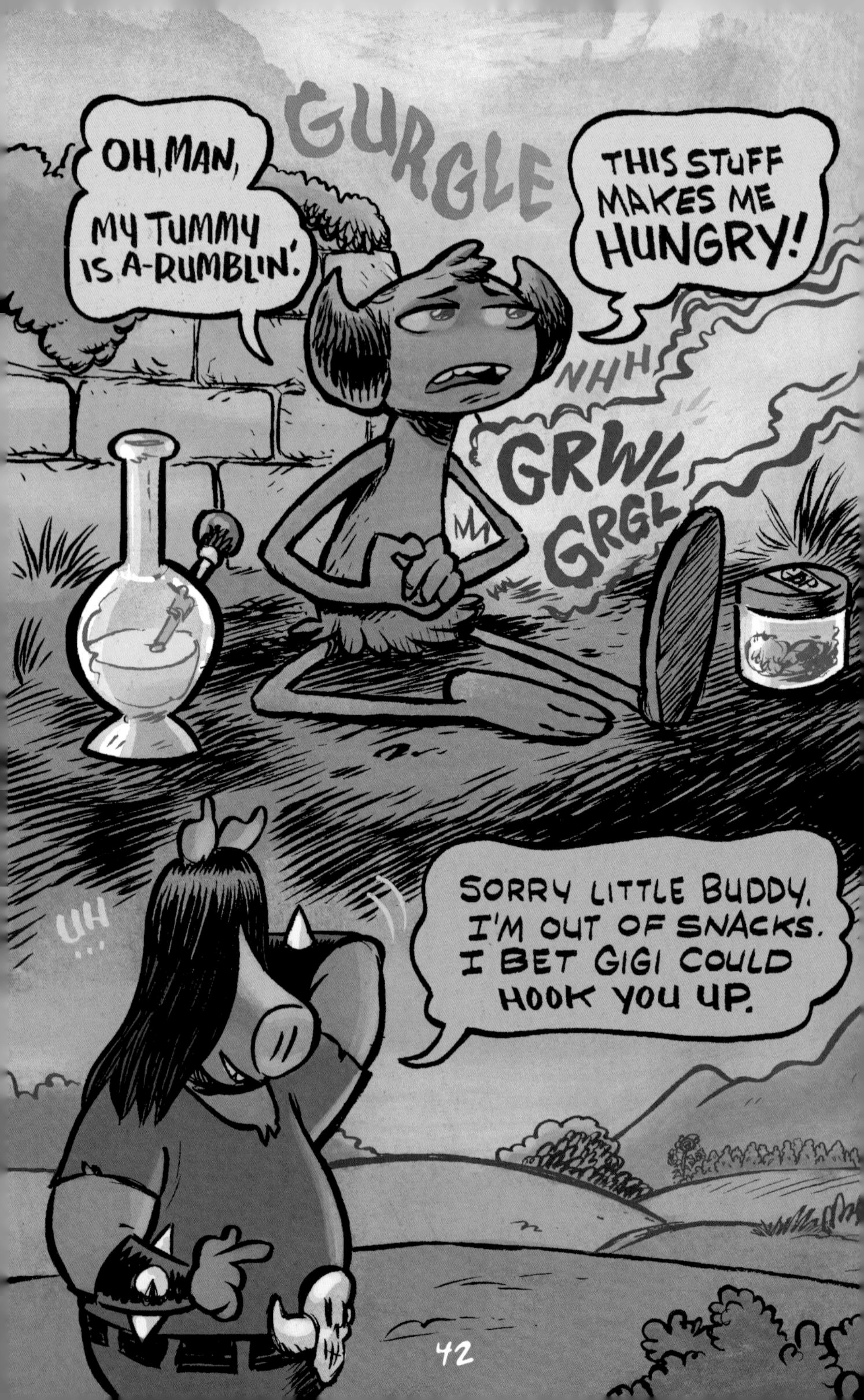
OH, MAN,
MY TUMMY IS A-RUMBLIN'.
GURGLE
THIS STUFF MAKES ME HUNGRY!
NHH
GRWL
GRGL
UH...
SORRY LITTLE BUDDY. I'M OUT OF SNACKS. I BET GIGI COULD HOOK YOU UP.

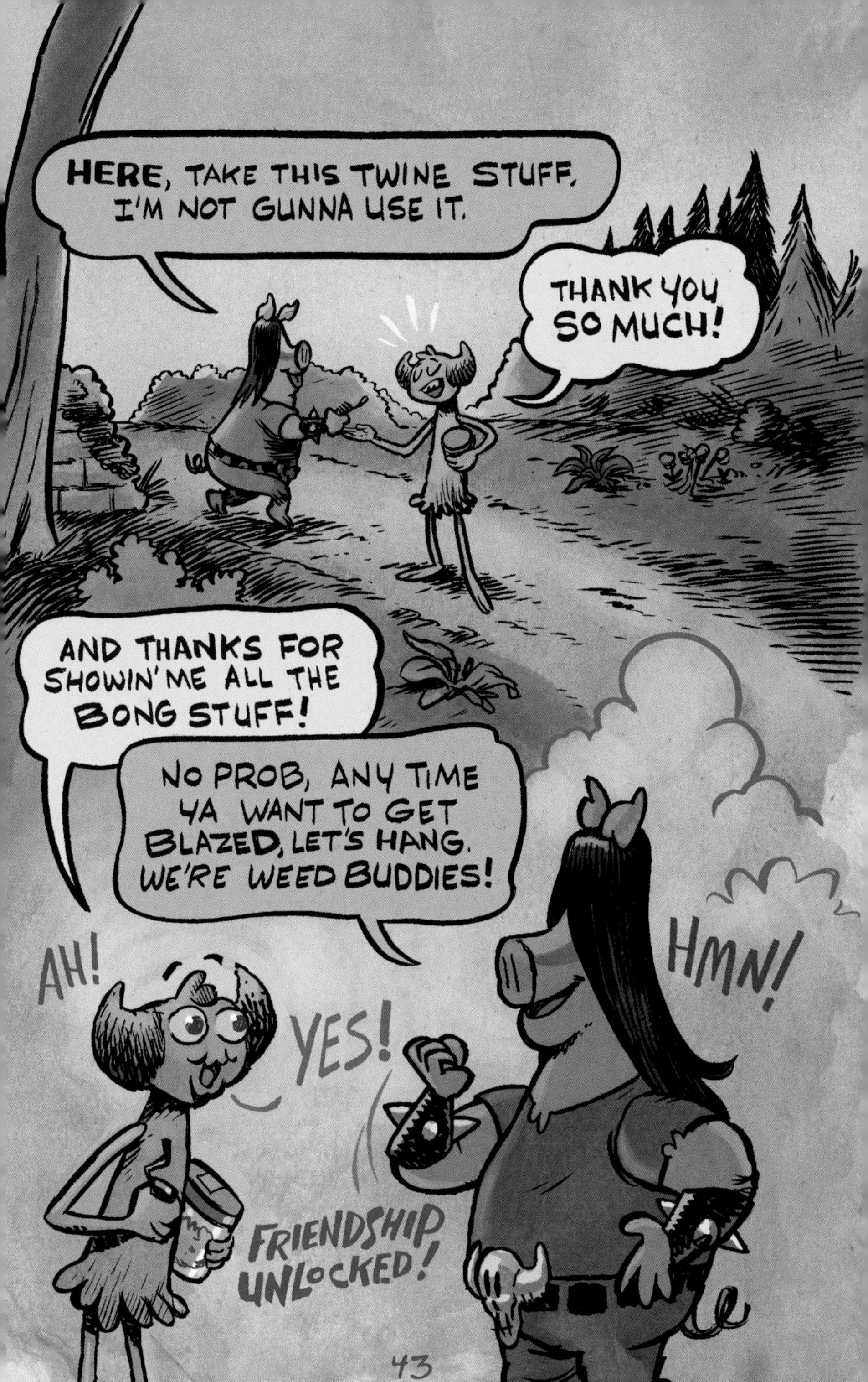
HERE, TAKE THIS TWINE STUFF. I'M NOT GUNNA USE IT.
THANK YOU SO MUCH!
AND THANKS FOR SHOWIN' ME ALL THE BONG STUFF!
NO PROB, ANY TIME YA WANT TO GET BLAZED, LET'S HANG. WE'RE WEED BUDDIES!
AH!
YES!
HMN!
FRIENDSHIP UNLOCKED!

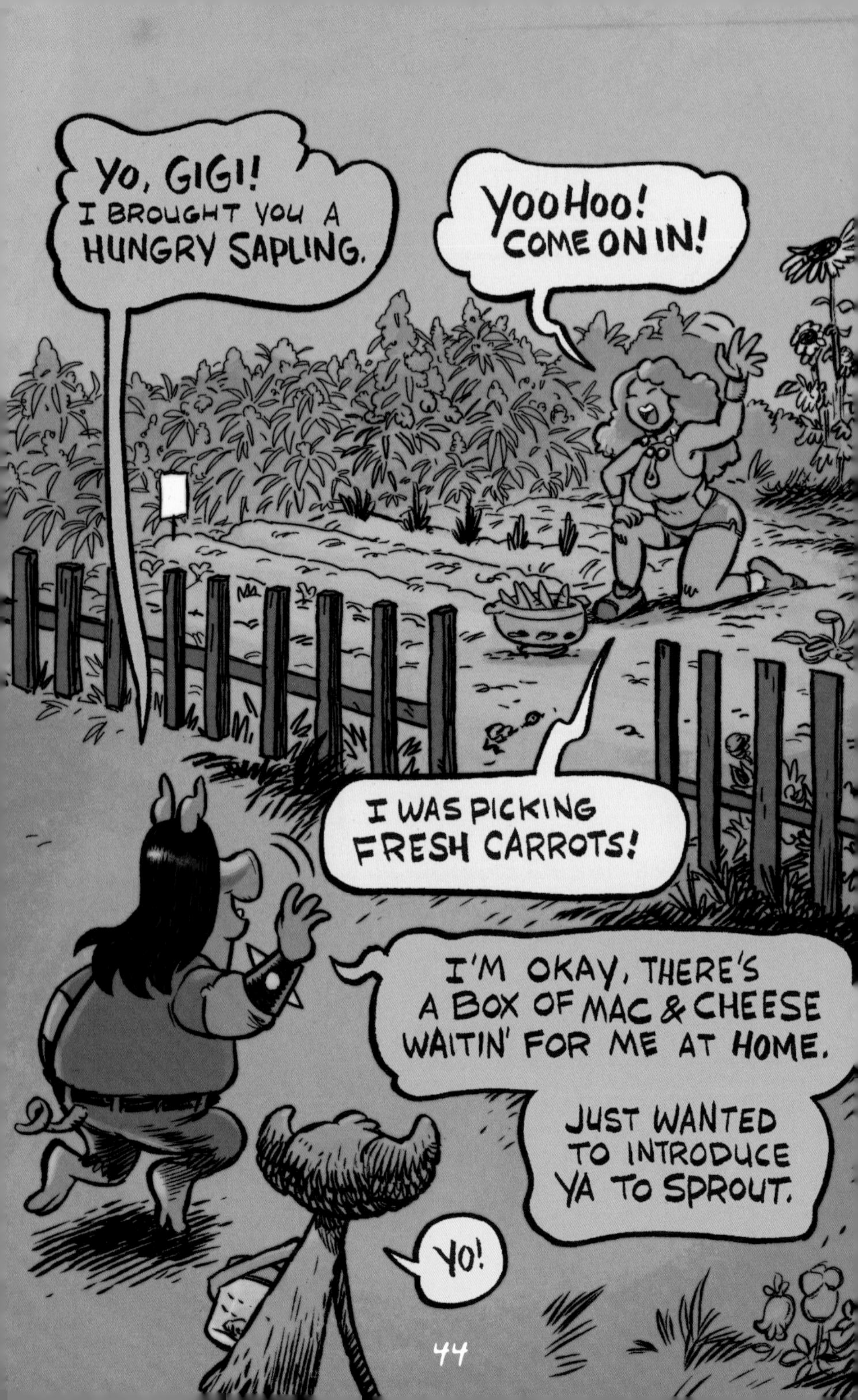
YO, GIGI! I BROUGHT YOU A HUNGRY SAPLING.
YOOHOO! COME ON IN!
I WAS PICKING FRESH CARROTS!
I'M OKAY, THERE'S A BOX OF MAC & CHEESE WAITIN' FOR ME AT HOME.
JUST WANTED TO INTRODUCE YA TO SPROUT.
YO!

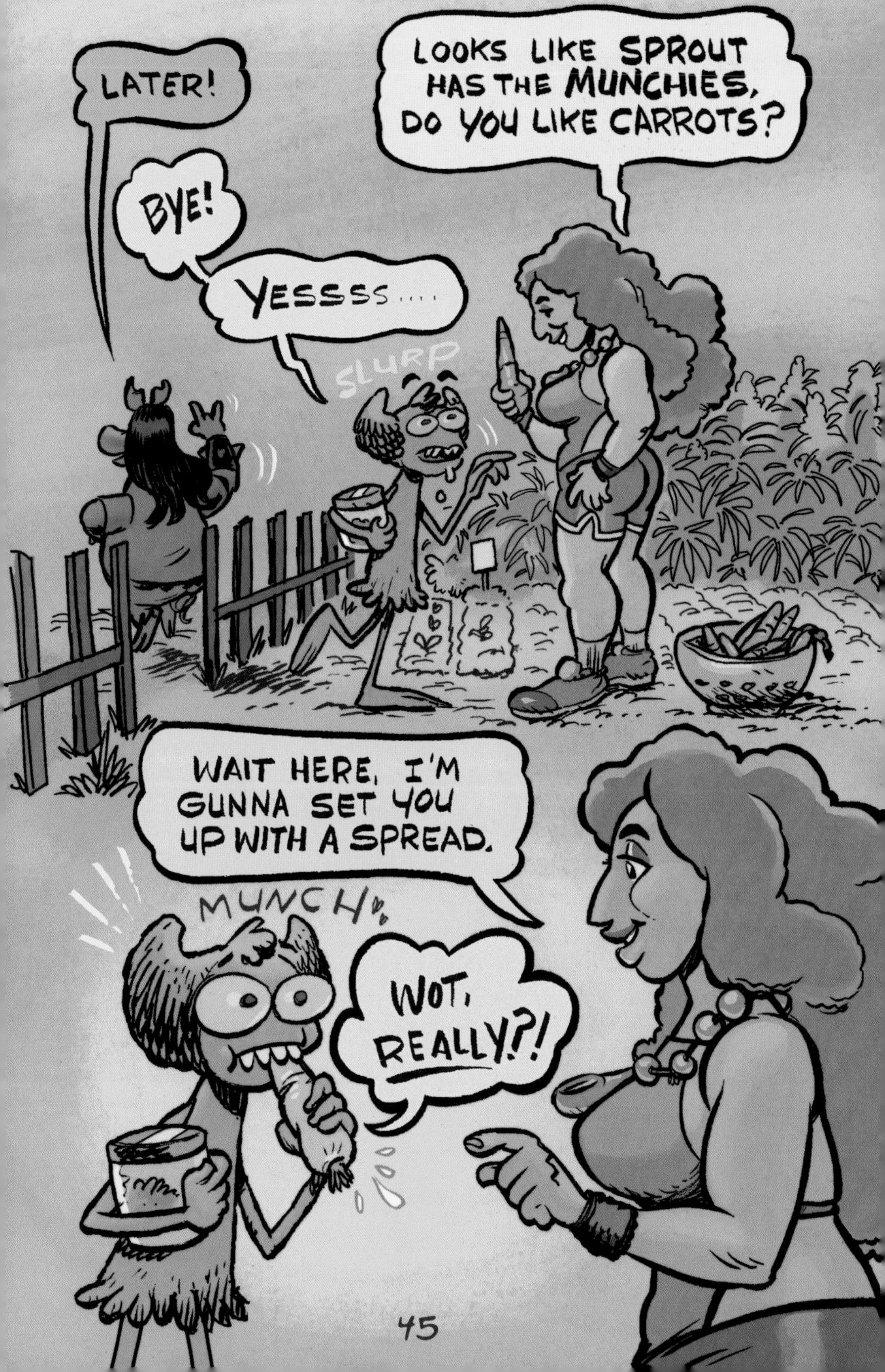
LOOKS LIKE SPROUT HAS THE MUNCHIES, DO YOU LIKE CARROTS?
LATER!
BYE!
YESSSS.....
SLURP
WAIT HERE, I'M GUNNA SET YOU UP WITH A SPREAD.
MUNCH
WOT, REALLY?!

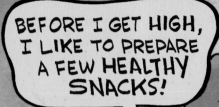

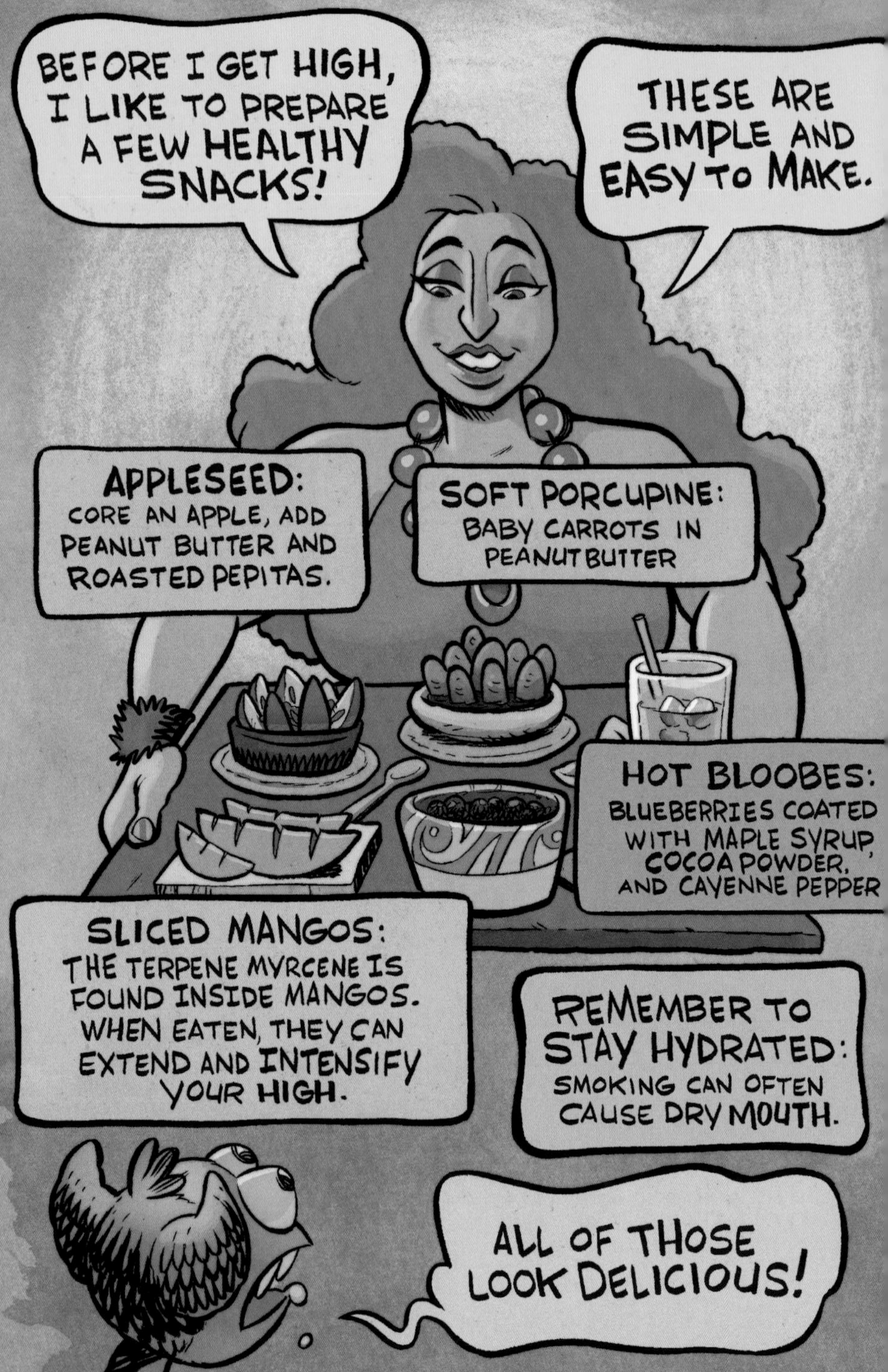

BEFORE I GET **HIGH**, I LIKE TO PREPARE A FEW **HEALTHY SNACKS!**

THESE ARE SIMPLE AND EASY TO MAKE.

APPLESEED: CORE AN APPLE, ADD PEANUT BUTTER AND ROASTED PEPITAS.

SOFT PORCUPINE: BABY CARROTS IN PEANUT BUTTER

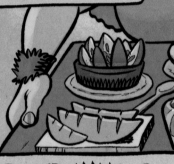

HOT BLOOBES: BLUEBERRIES COATED WITH MAPLE SYRUP, COCOA POWDER, AND CAYENNE PEPPER

SLICED MANGOS: THE TERPENE MYRCENE IS FOUND INSIDE MANGOS. WHEN EATEN, THEY CAN EXTEND AND **INTENSIFY** YOUR **HIGH**.

REMEMBER TO STAY HYDRATED: SMOKING CAN OFTEN CAUSE DRY MOUTH.

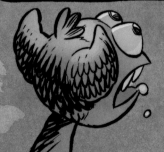

ALL OF THOSE LOOK **DELICIOUS!**

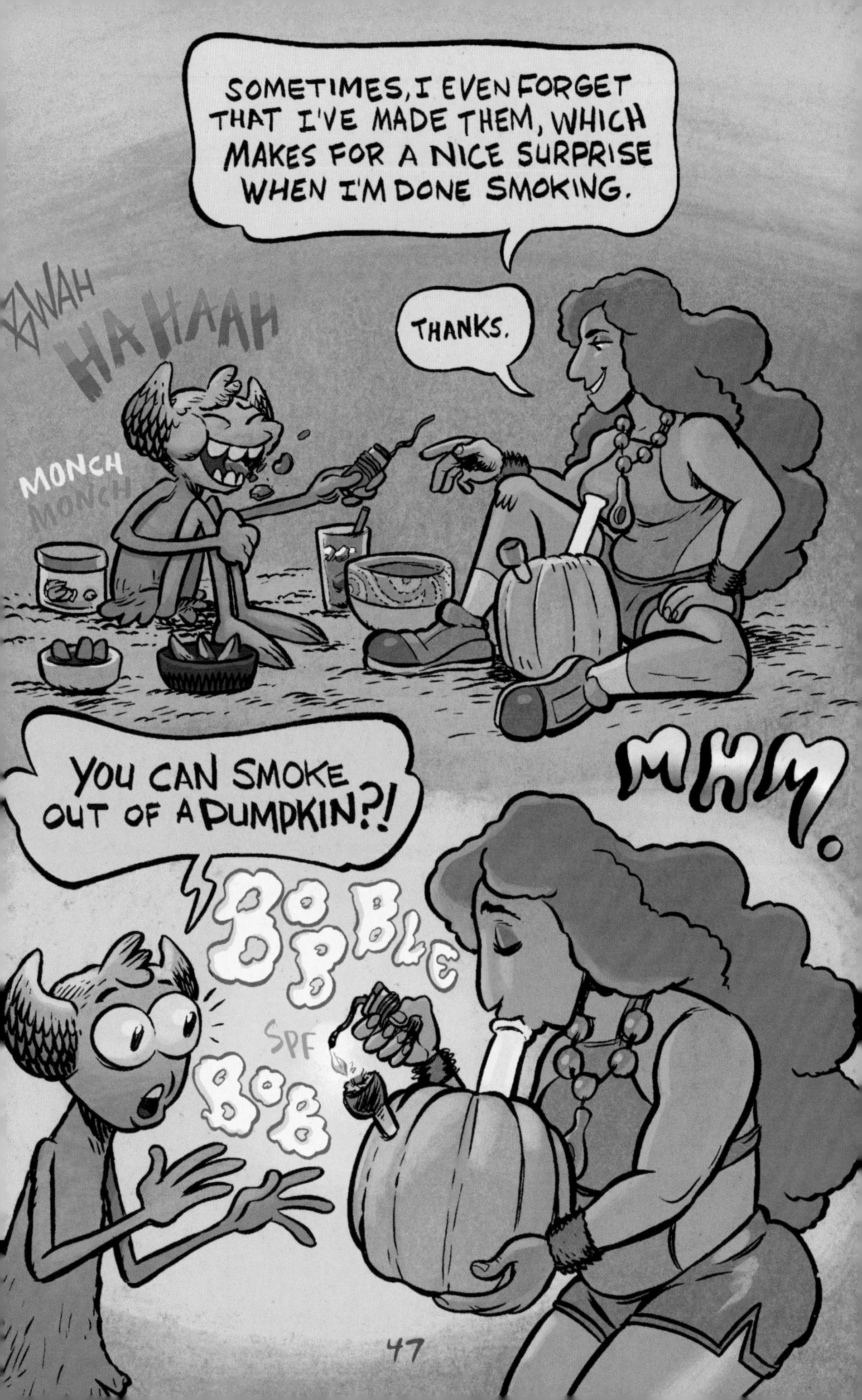
SOMETIMES, I EVEN FORGET THAT I'VE MADE THEM, WHICH MAKES FOR A NICE SURPRISE WHEN I'M DONE SMOKING.
BWAH HA HAAAH
THANKS.
MONCH
MONCH
YOU CAN SMOKE OUT OF A PUMPKIN?!
MHM.
BOBBLE
SPF
BOB

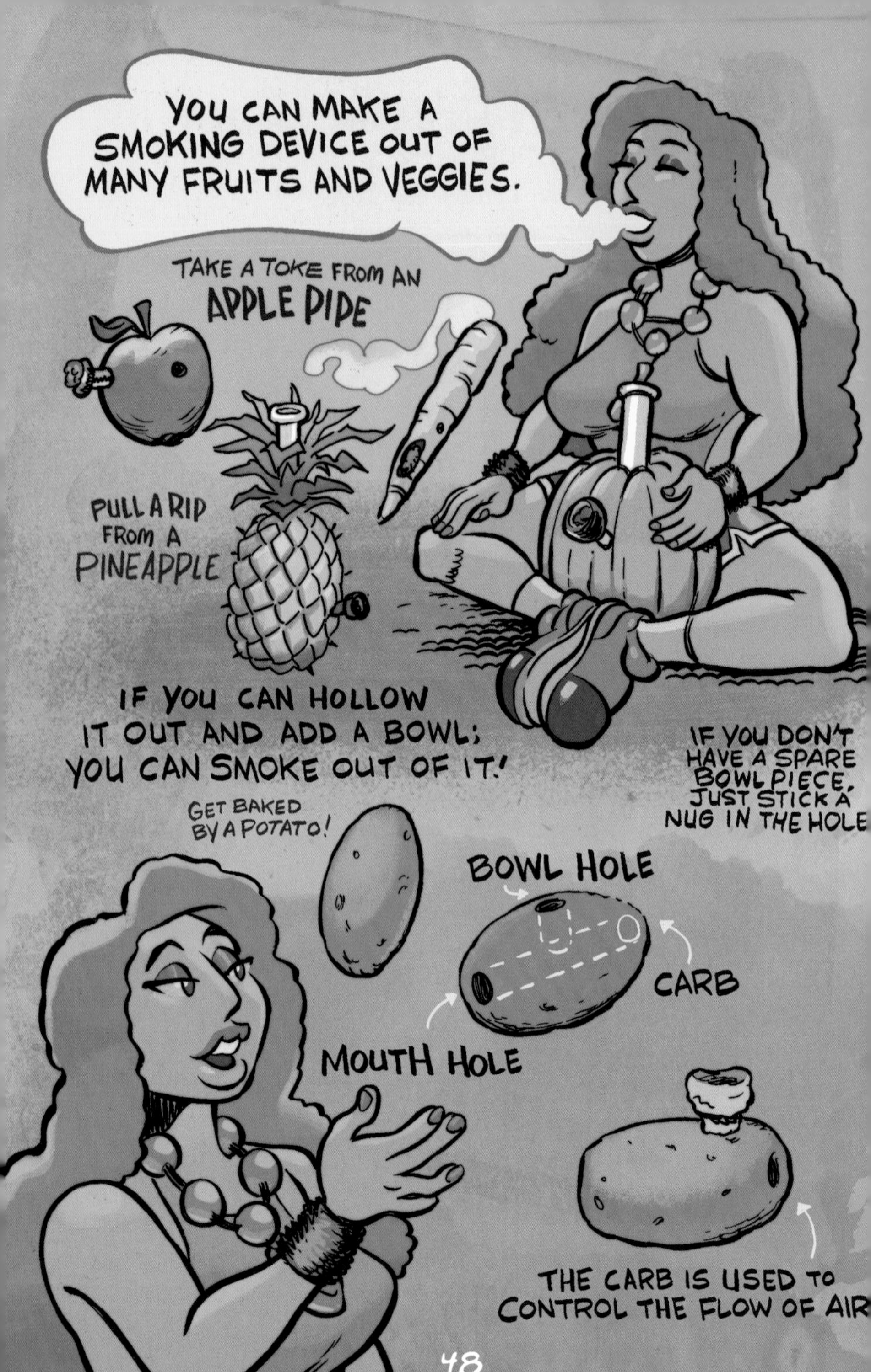
YOU CAN MAKE A SMOKING DEVICE OUT OF MANY FRUITS AND VEGGIES.
TAKE A TOKE FROM AN APPLE PIPE
PULL A RIP FROM A PINEAPPLE
IF YOU CAN HOLLOW IT OUT AND ADD A BOWL; YOU CAN SMOKE OUT OF IT!
IF YOU DON'T HAVE A SPARE BOWL PIECE, JUST STICK A NUG IN THE HOLE
GET BAKED BY A POTATO!
BOWL HOLE
CARB
MOUTH HOLE
THE CARB IS USED TO CONTROL THE FLOW OF AIR

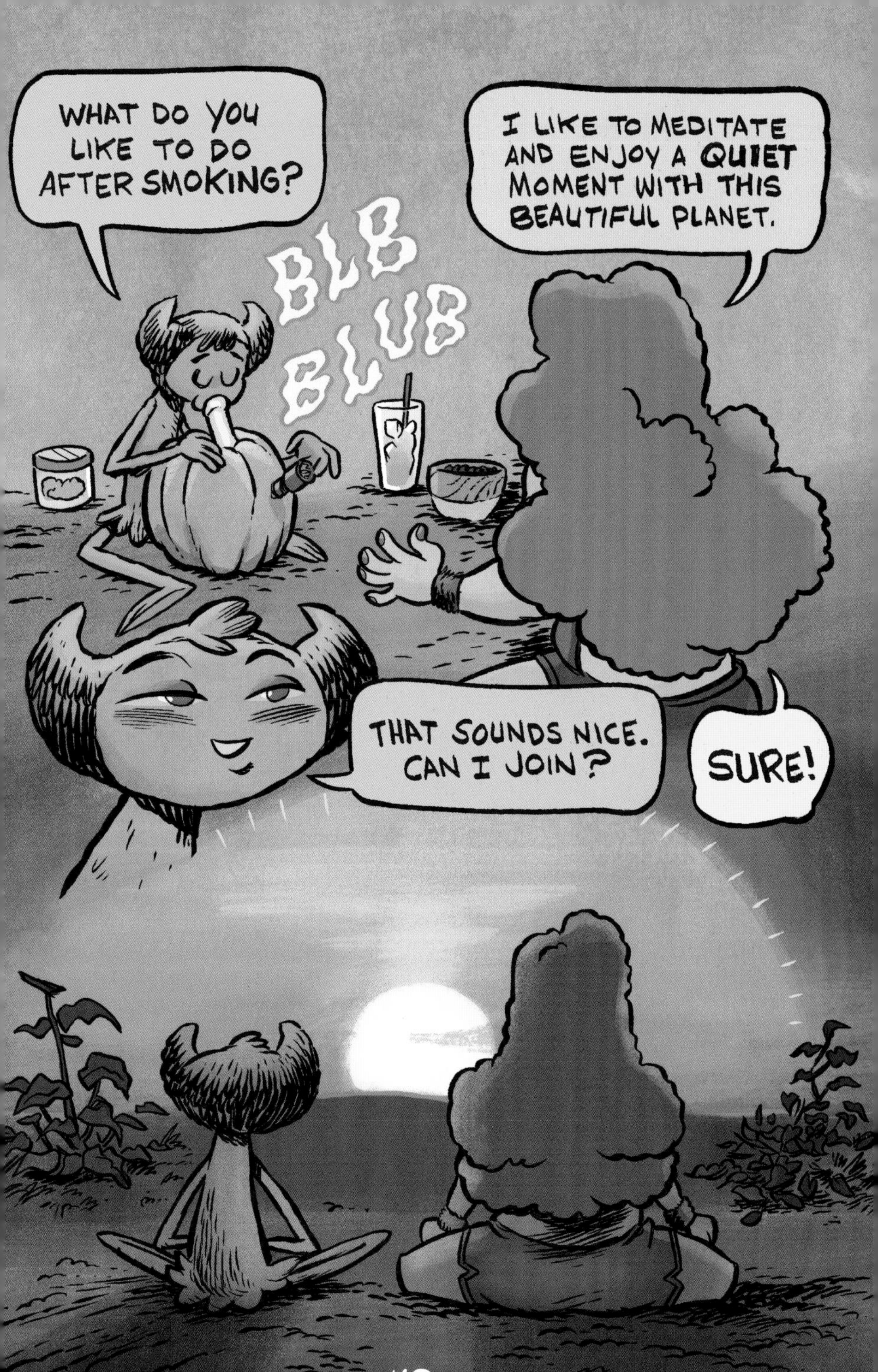
WHAT DO YOU LIKE TO DO AFTER SMOKING?
I LIKE TO MEDITATE AND ENJOY A QUIET MOMENT WITH THIS BEAUTIFUL PLANET.
BLB BLUB
THAT SOUNDS NICE. CAN I JOIN?
SURE!

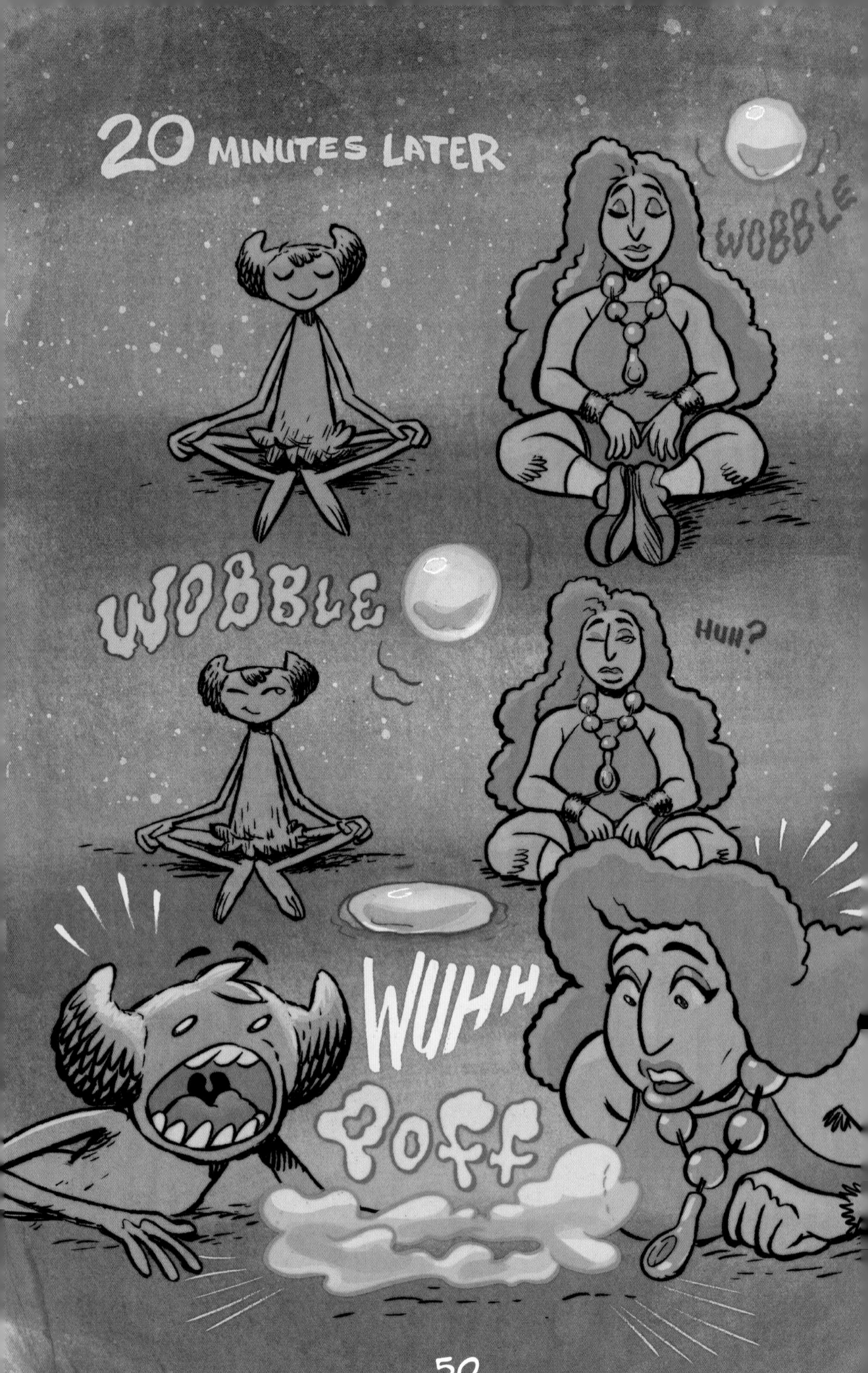
20 MINUTES LATER
WOBBLE
WOBBLE
HUH?
WUHH
POFF

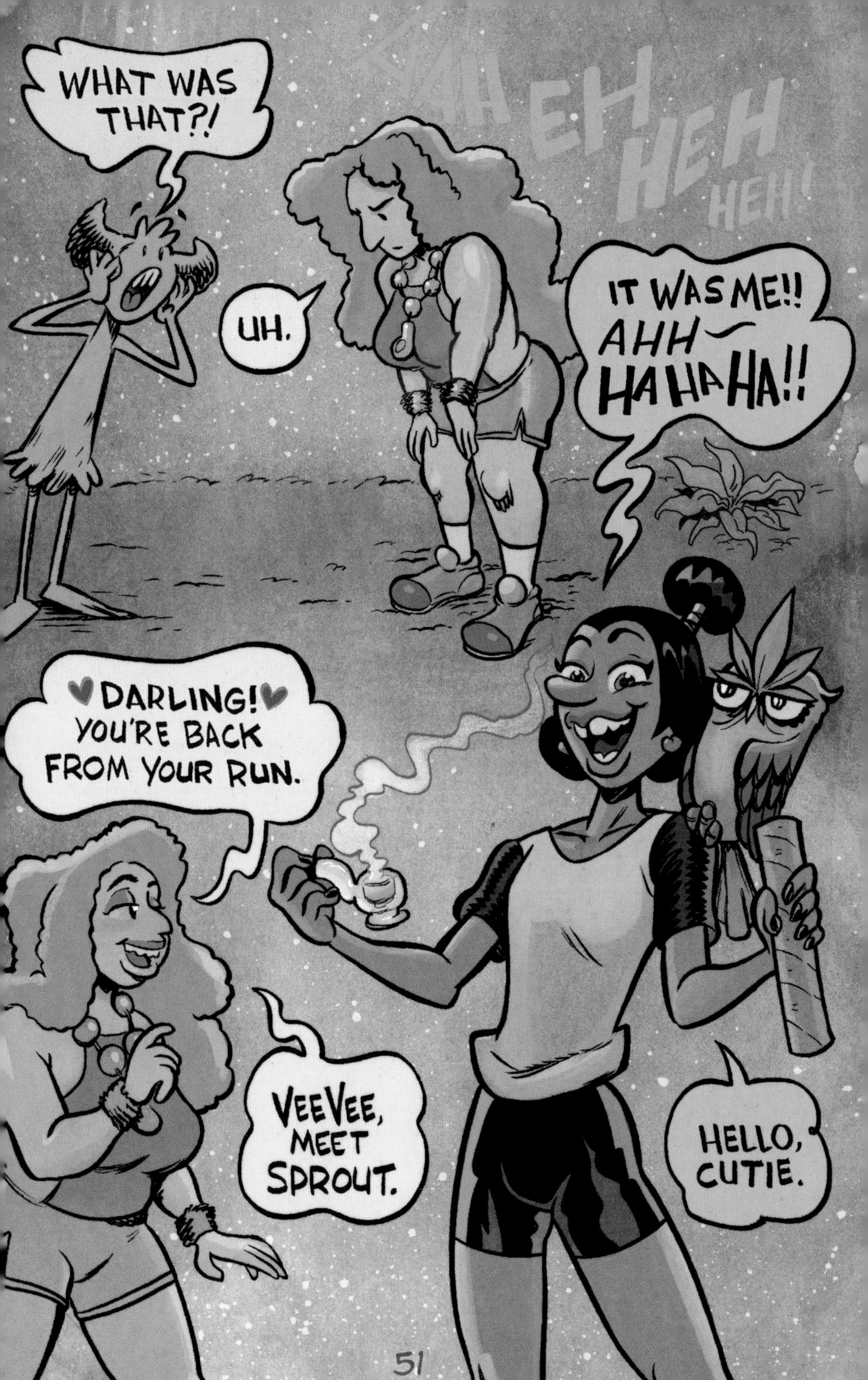
WHAT WAS THAT?!
HEH HEH HEH!
UH.
IT WAS ME!! AHH~ HAHAHA!!
DARLING! YOU'RE BACK FROM YOUR RUN.
VEEVEE, MEET SPROUT.
HELLO, CUTIE.

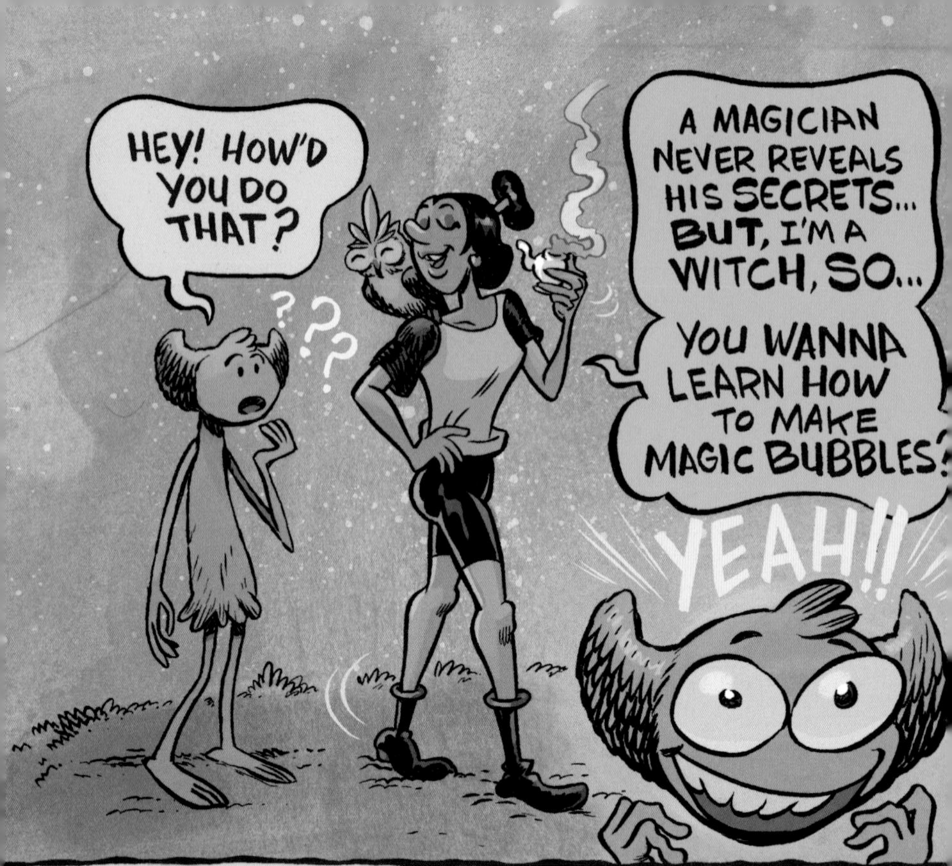
HEY! HOW'D YOU DO THAT?
A MAGICIAN NEVER REVEALS HIS SECRETS... BUT, I'M A WITCH, SO...
YOU WANNA LEARN HOW TO MAKE MAGIC BUBBLES?
YEAH!!

WHAT YOU NEED TO MAKE MAGIC BUBBLES:

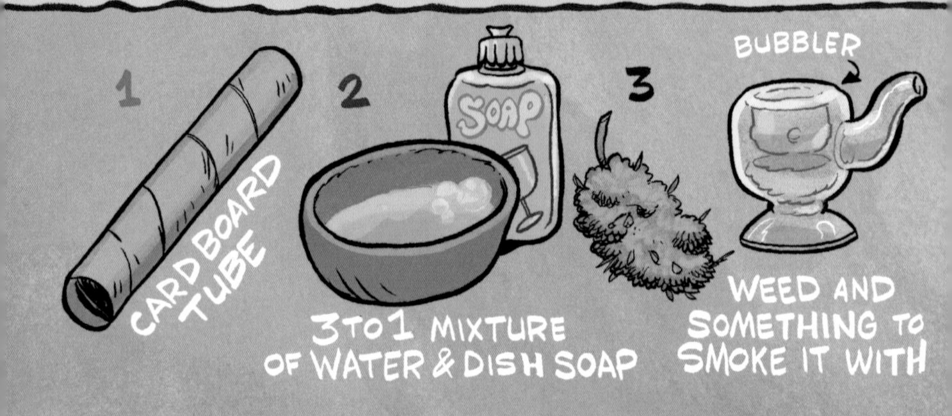
1
CARDBOARD TUBE
2
SOAP
3 TO 1 MIXTURE OF WATER & DISH SOAP
3
BUBBLER
WEED AND SOMETHING TO SMOKE IT WITH

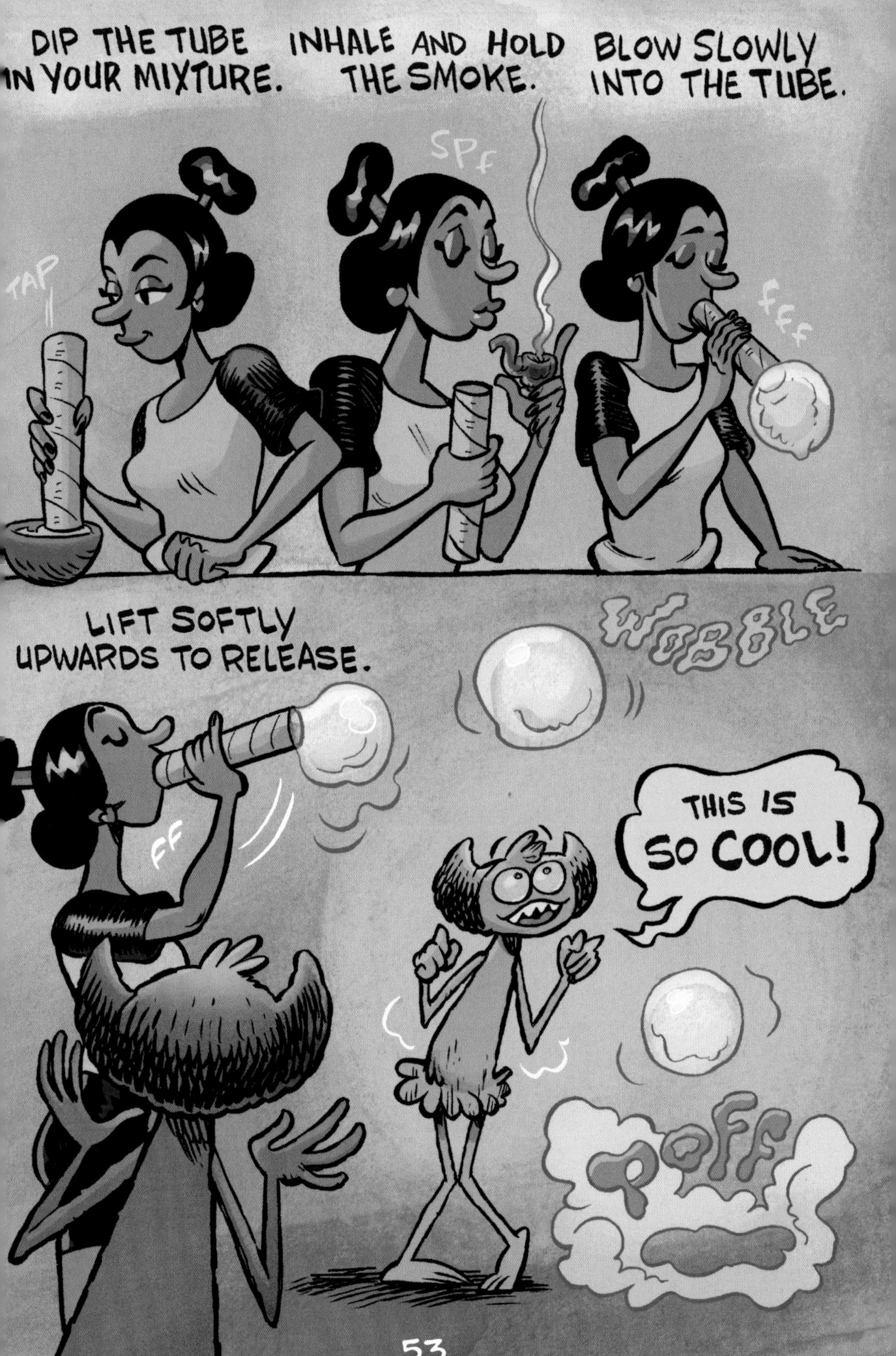
DIP THE TUBE IN YOUR MIXTURE.
TAP
INHALE AND HOLD THE SMOKE.
SPF
BLOW SLOWLY INTO THE TUBE.
FFF
LIFT SOFTLY UPWARDS TO RELEASE.
FF
WOBBLE
THIS IS SO COOL!
POFF

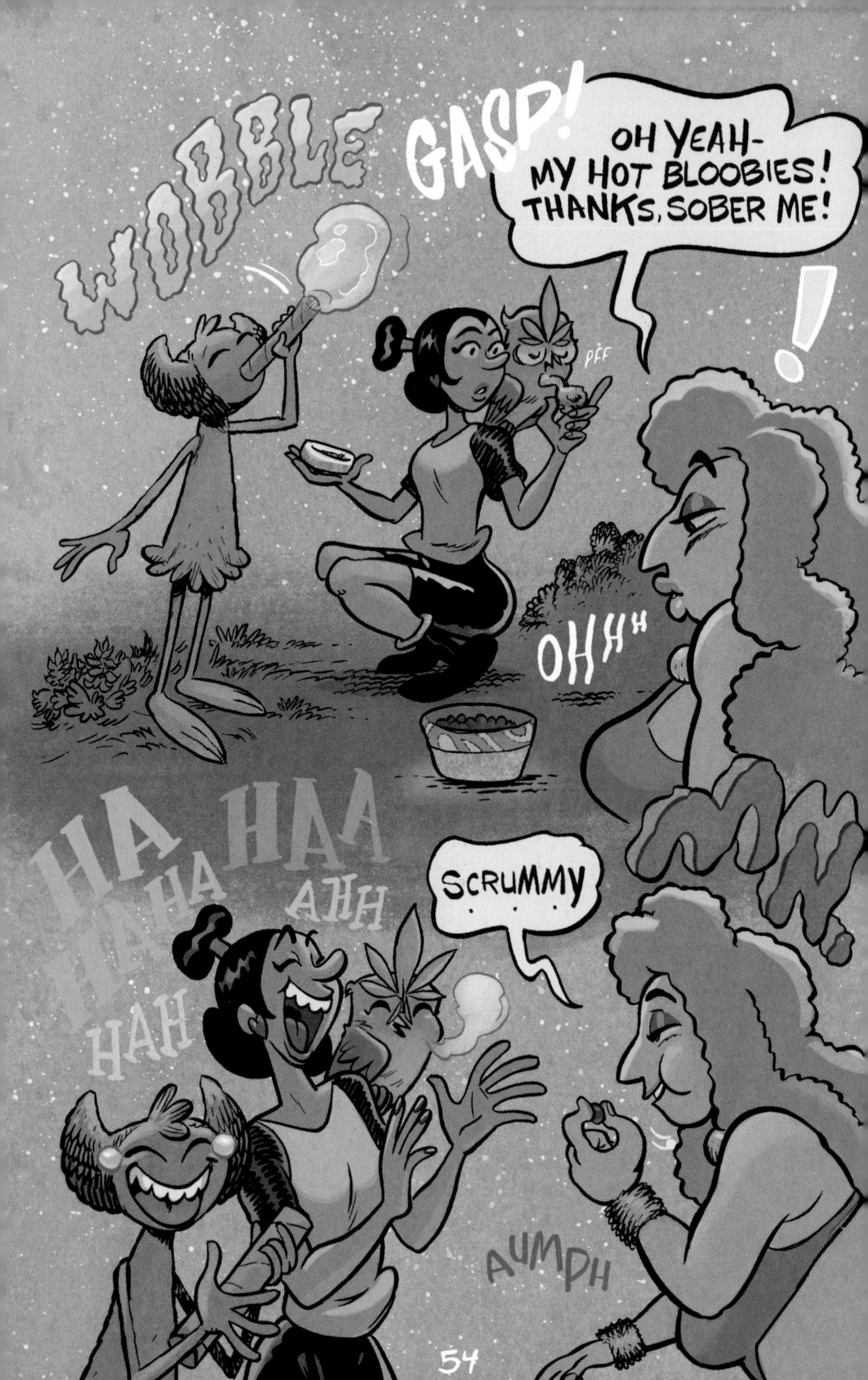
WOBBLE
GASP!
OH YEAH-
MY HOT BLOOBIES!
THANKS, SOBER ME!
PFF
!
OHHH
MMM
HA HA HAA HA
AHH
HAH
SCRUMMY...
AUMPH

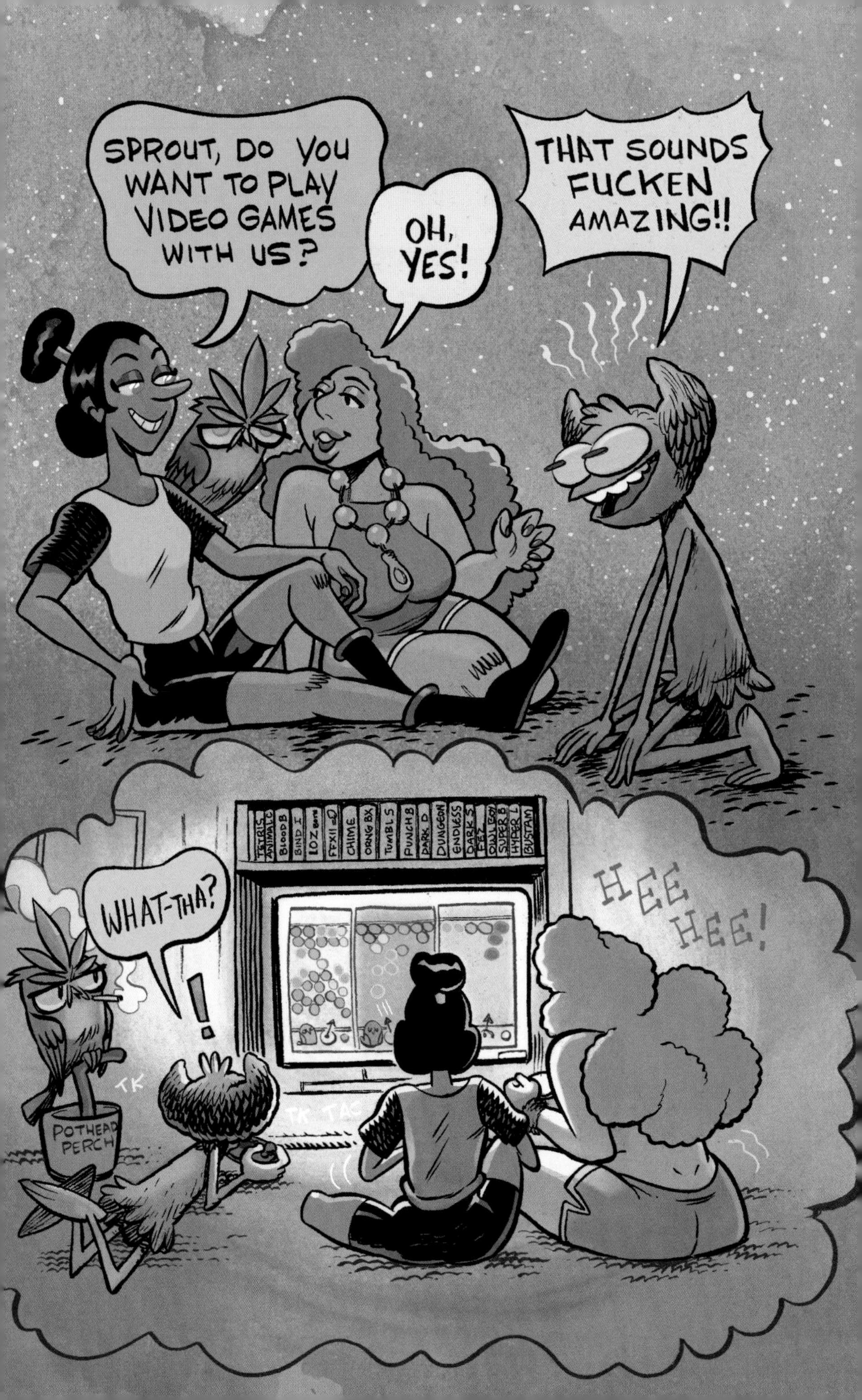
SPROUT, DO YOU WANT TO PLAY VIDEO GAMES WITH US?
OH, YES!
THAT SOUNDS FUCKEN AMAZING!!
WHAT-THA?
!
HEE HEE!
TK
TK TAC
POTHEAD PERCH

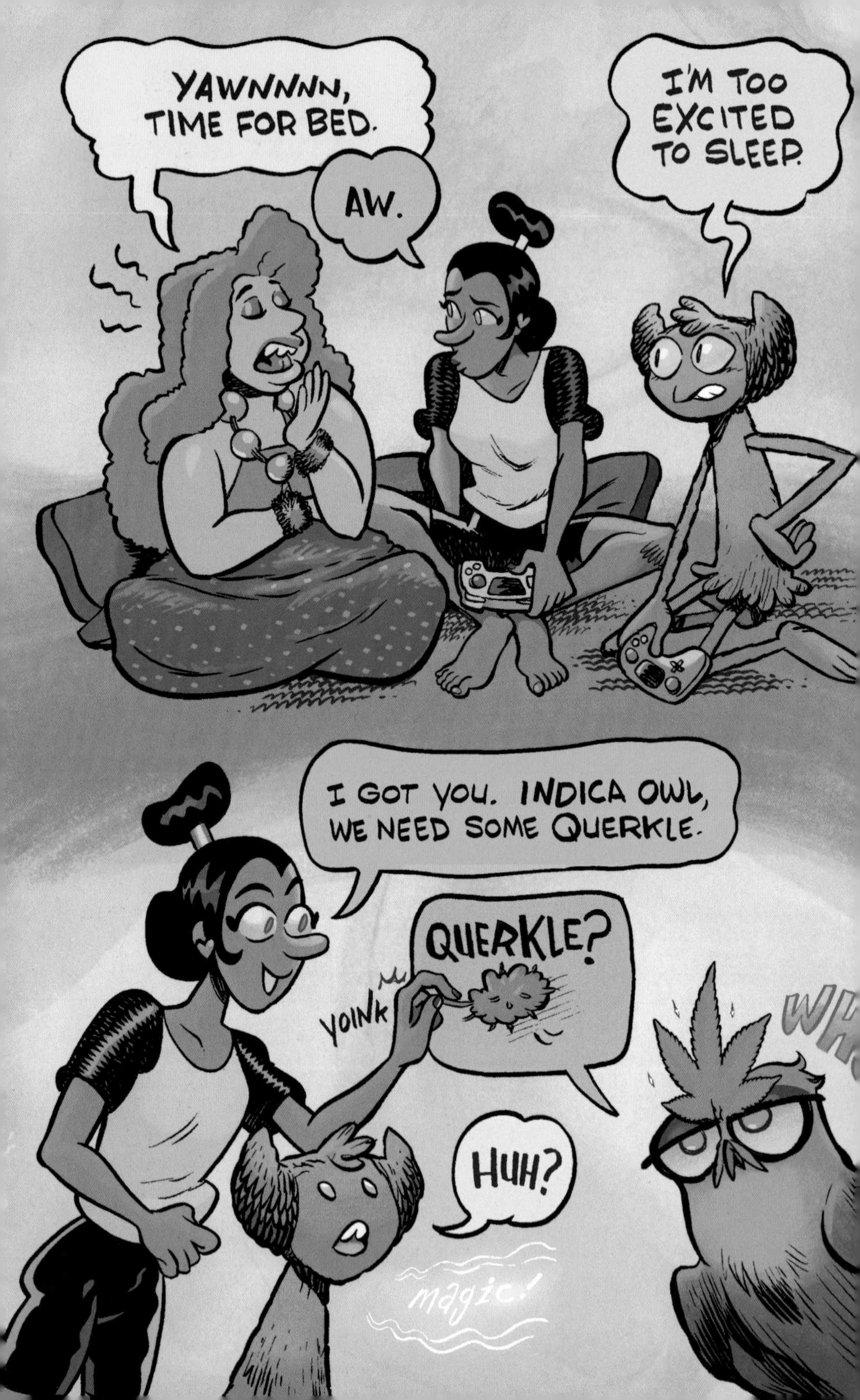
YAWNNNN, TIME FOR BED.
AW.
I'M TOO EXCITED TO SLEEP.
I GOT YOU. INDICA OWL, WE NEED SOME QUERKLE.
QUERKLE?
YOINK
HUH?
magic!

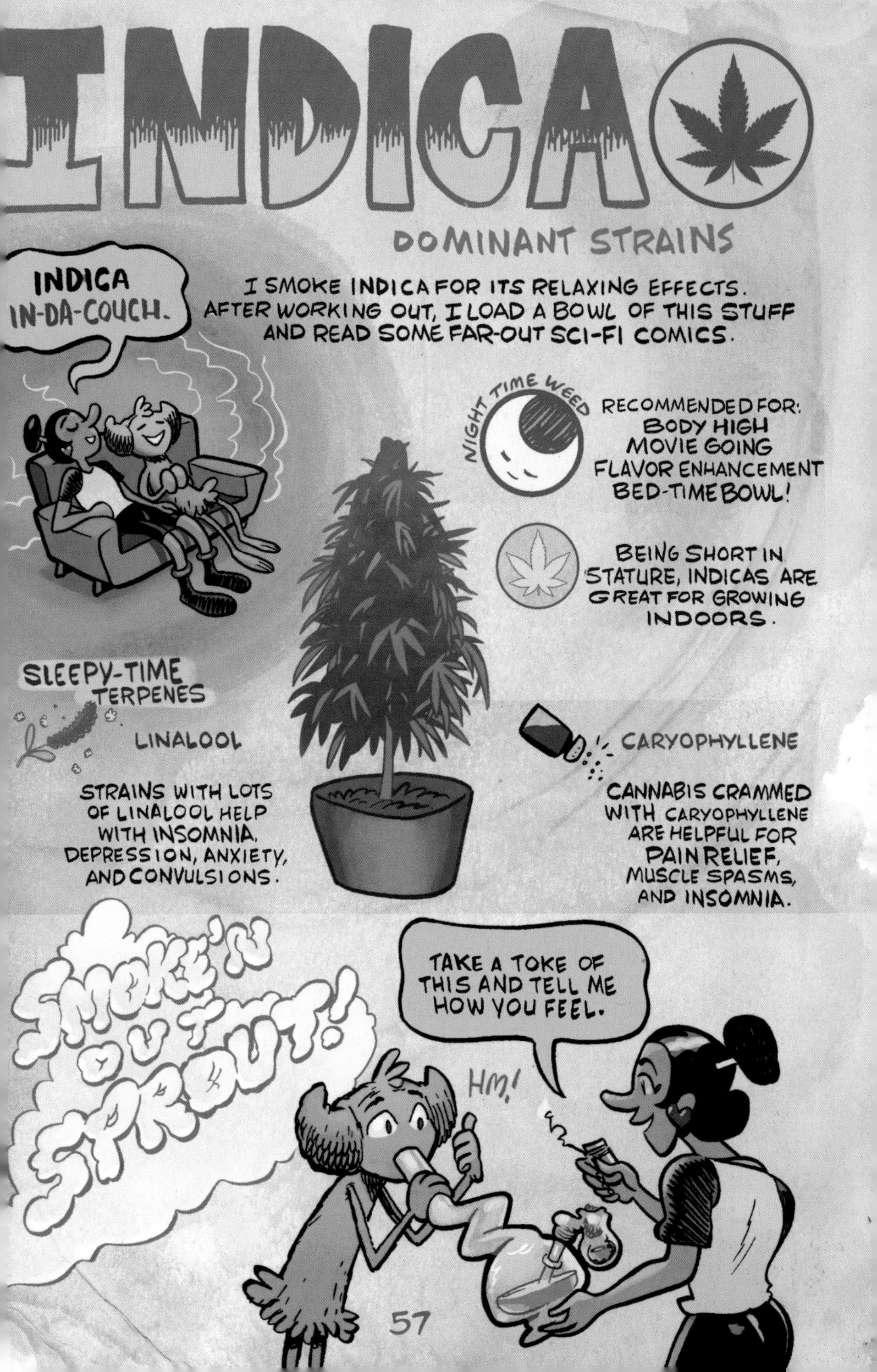
INDICA
DOMINANT STRAINS
INDICA IN-DA-COUCH.
I SMOKE INDICA FOR ITS RELAXING EFFECTS. AFTER WORKING OUT, I LOAD A BOWL OF THIS STUFF AND READ SOME FAR-OUT SCI-FI COMICS.
NIGHT TIME WEED
RECOMMENDED FOR:
BODY HIGH
MOVIE GOING
FLAVOR ENHANCEMENT
BED-TIME BOWL!
BEING SHORT IN STATURE, INDICAS ARE GREAT FOR GROWING INDOORS.
SLEEPY-TIME TERPENES
LINALOOL
STRAINS WITH LOTS OF LINALOOL HELP WITH INSOMNIA, DEPRESSION, ANXIETY, AND CONVULSIONS.
CARYOPHYLLENE
CANNABIS CRAMMED WITH CARYOPHYLLENE ARE HELPFUL FOR PAIN RELIEF, MUSCLE SPASMS, AND INSOMNIA.
SMOKE'N OUT SPROUT!
TAKE A TOKE OF THIS AND TELL ME HOW YOU FEEL.
HM!

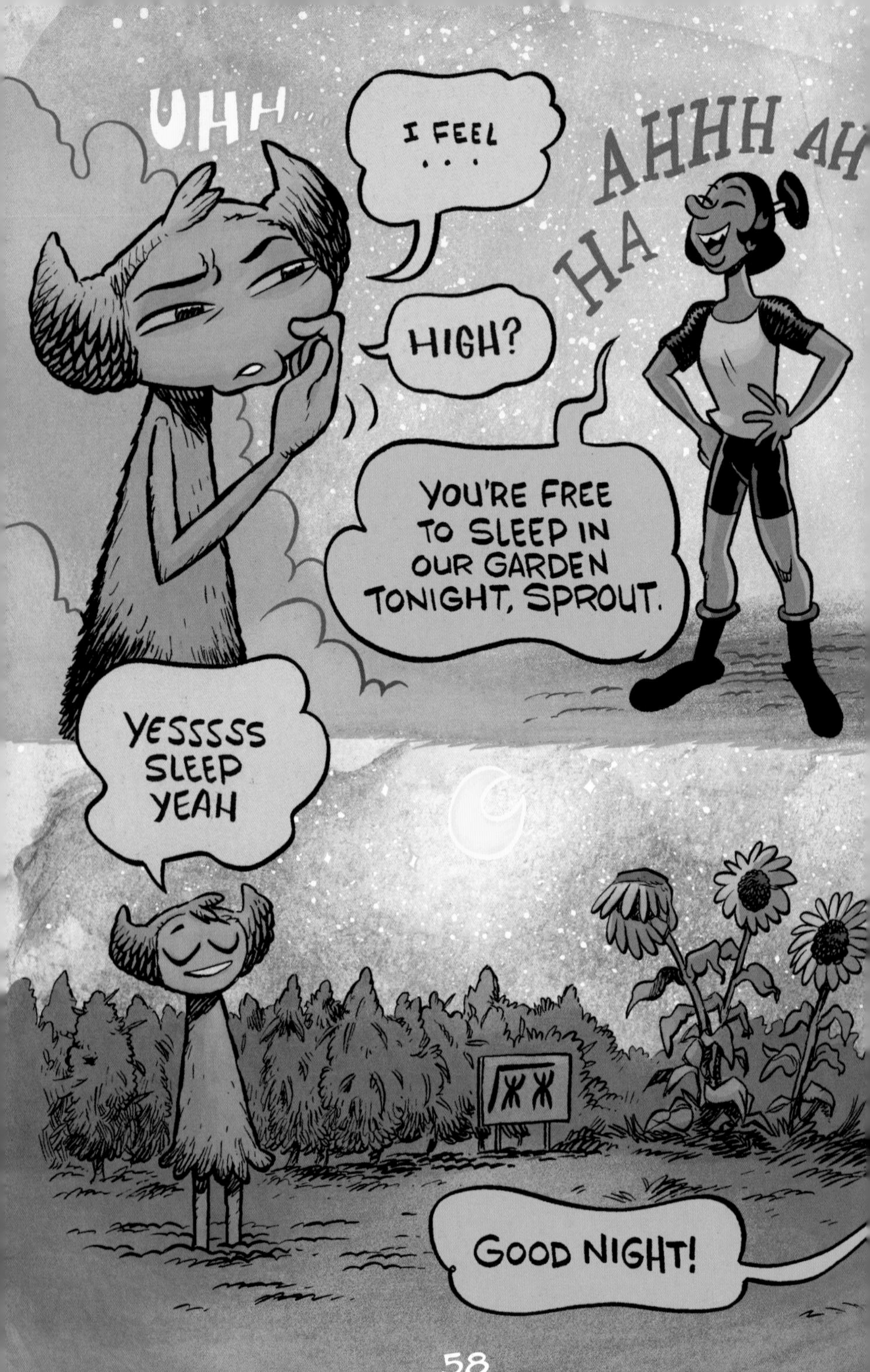
UHH...
I FEEL . . .
HIGH?
AHHH AH HA
YOU'RE FREE TO SLEEP IN OUR GARDEN TONIGHT, SPROUT.
YESSSSS SLEEP YEAH
GOOD NIGHT!

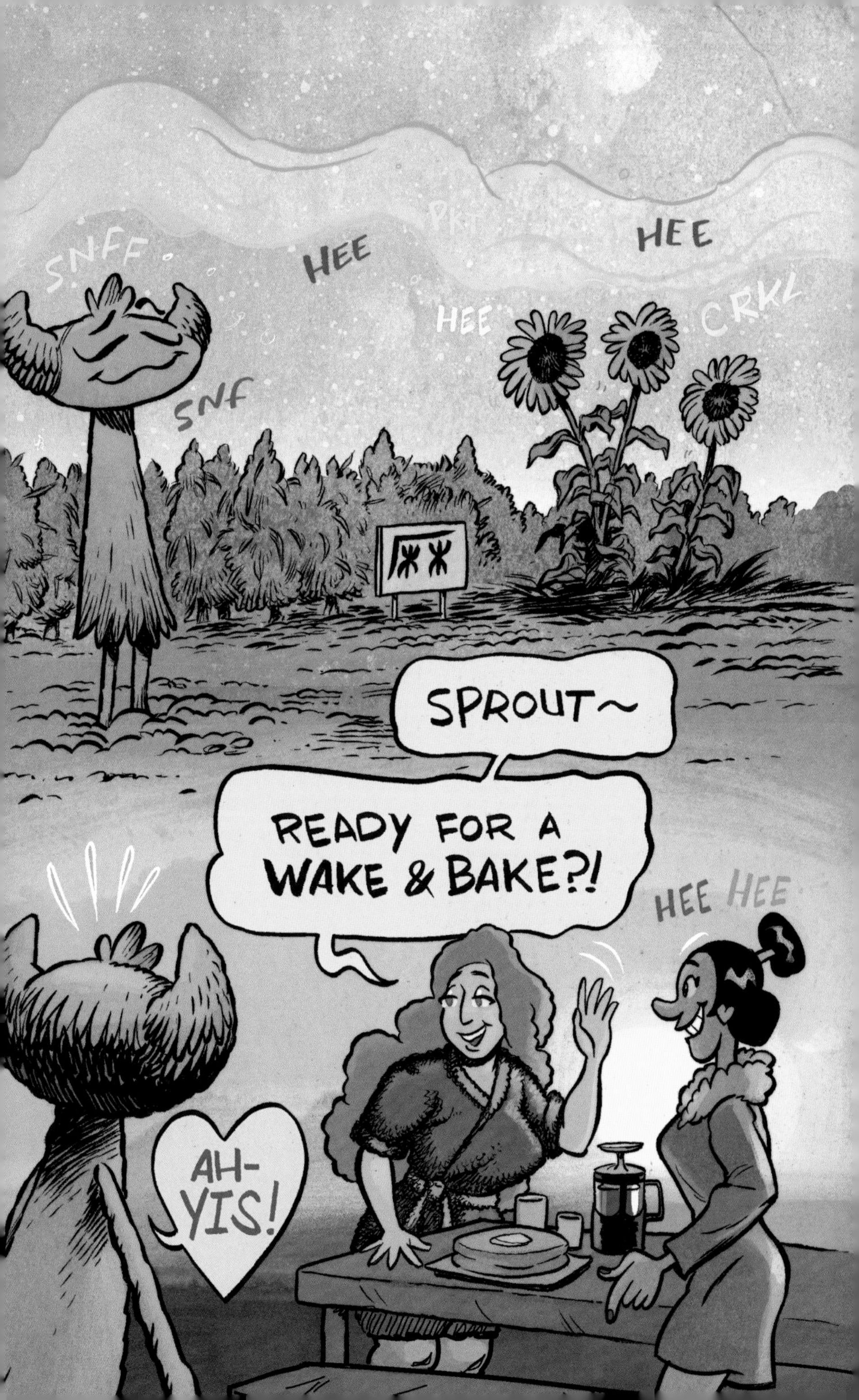
SNFF
HEE
PKT
HEE
HEE
CRKL
SNF
SPROUT~
READY FOR A WAKE & BAKE?!
HEE HEE
AH-YIS!

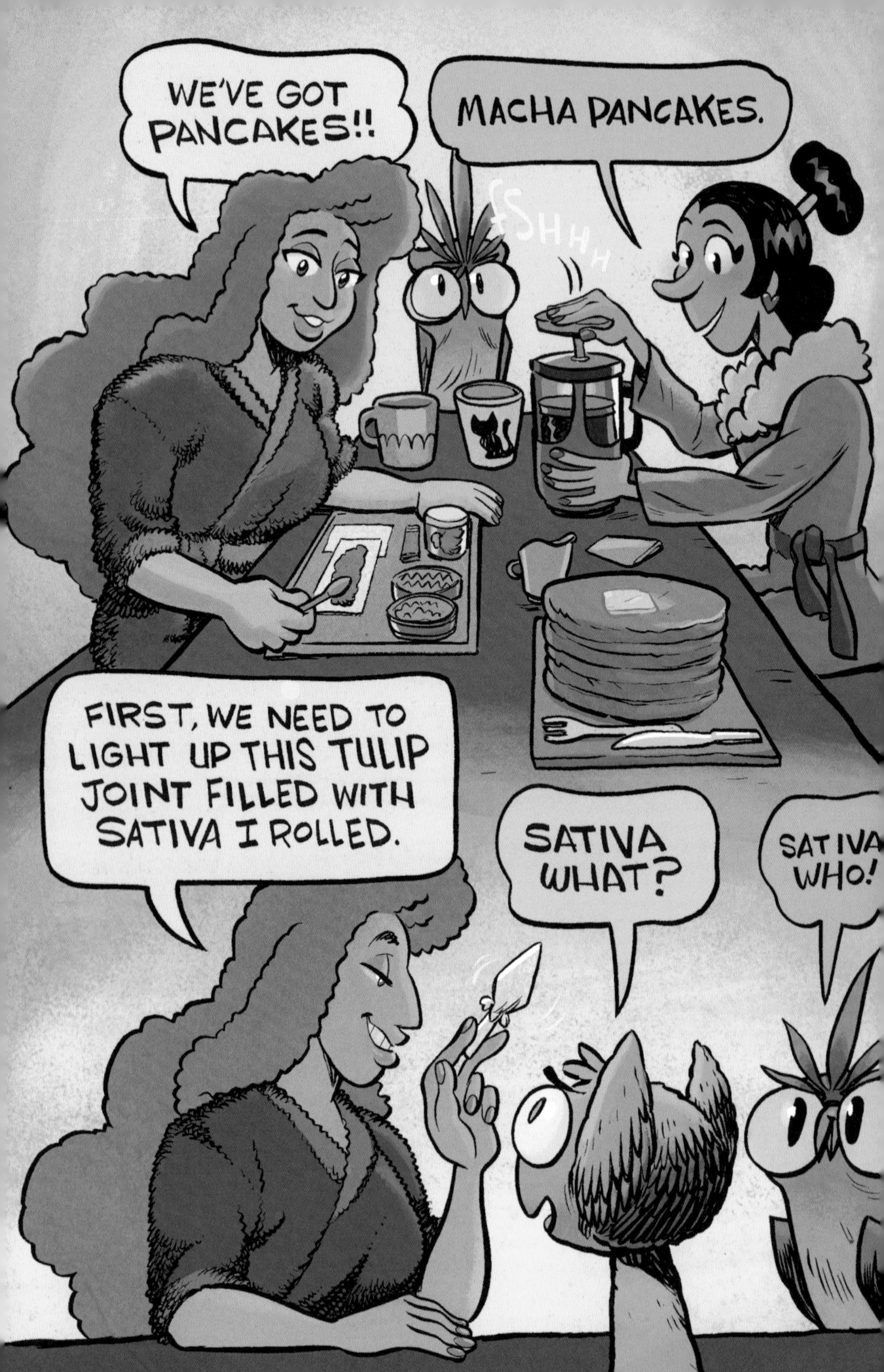
WE'VE GOT PANCAKES!!
MACHA PANCAKES.
FSHHHH
FIRST, WE NEED TO LIGHT UP THIS TULIP JOINT FILLED WITH SATIVA I ROLLED.
SATIVA WHAT?
SATIVA WHO!

SATIVA DOMINANT STRAIN

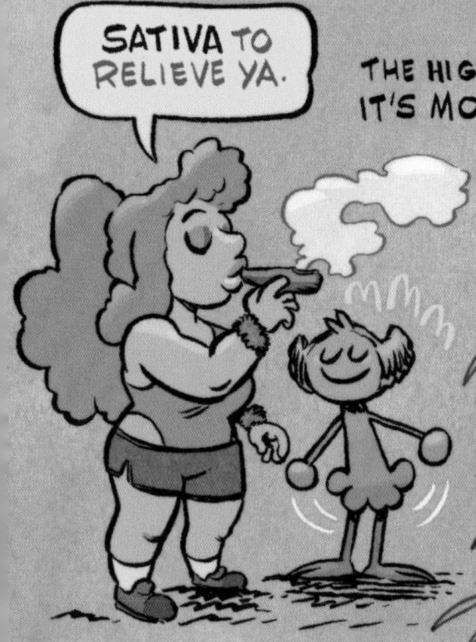
SATIVA TO RELIEVE YA.
MMM

THE HIGH I GET FROM SATIVA IS VERY ENERGIZING. IT'S MORE CEREBRAL AND KEEPS ME ON TASK WHILE I TEND TO MY GARDEN.

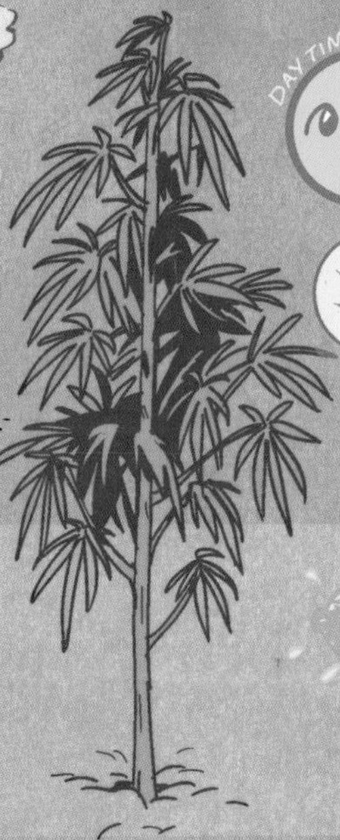

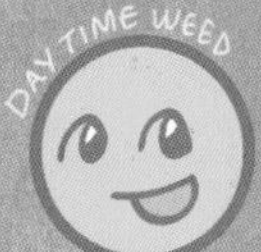
DAY TIME WEED

RECCOMENDED FOR:
- DRAWING
- LONG WALKS
- PLAYING GAMES
- SOCIAL GATHERINGS

HARDER TO GROW, BECAUSE OF THEIR HEIGHT AND LONG GROWTH PHASE. PRIMARILY GROWN OUTDOORS.

TERPENES TO WATCH FOR:

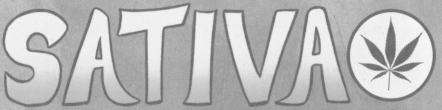

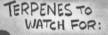

HUMULENE

HEAPS OF THESE HOPS-LIKE TERPENES CAN ACTUALLY HELP SUPPRESS APPETITE.

LIMONENE

CANNABIS WITH LOADS OF LIMONENE HELPS LIFT YOUR MOOD AND LOWER YOUR STRESS.

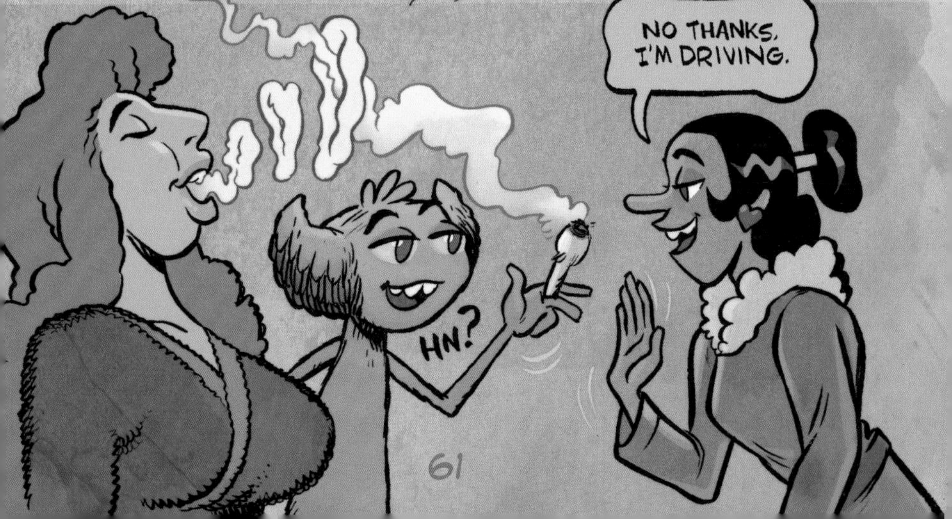
NO THANKS, I'M DRIVING.
HN?

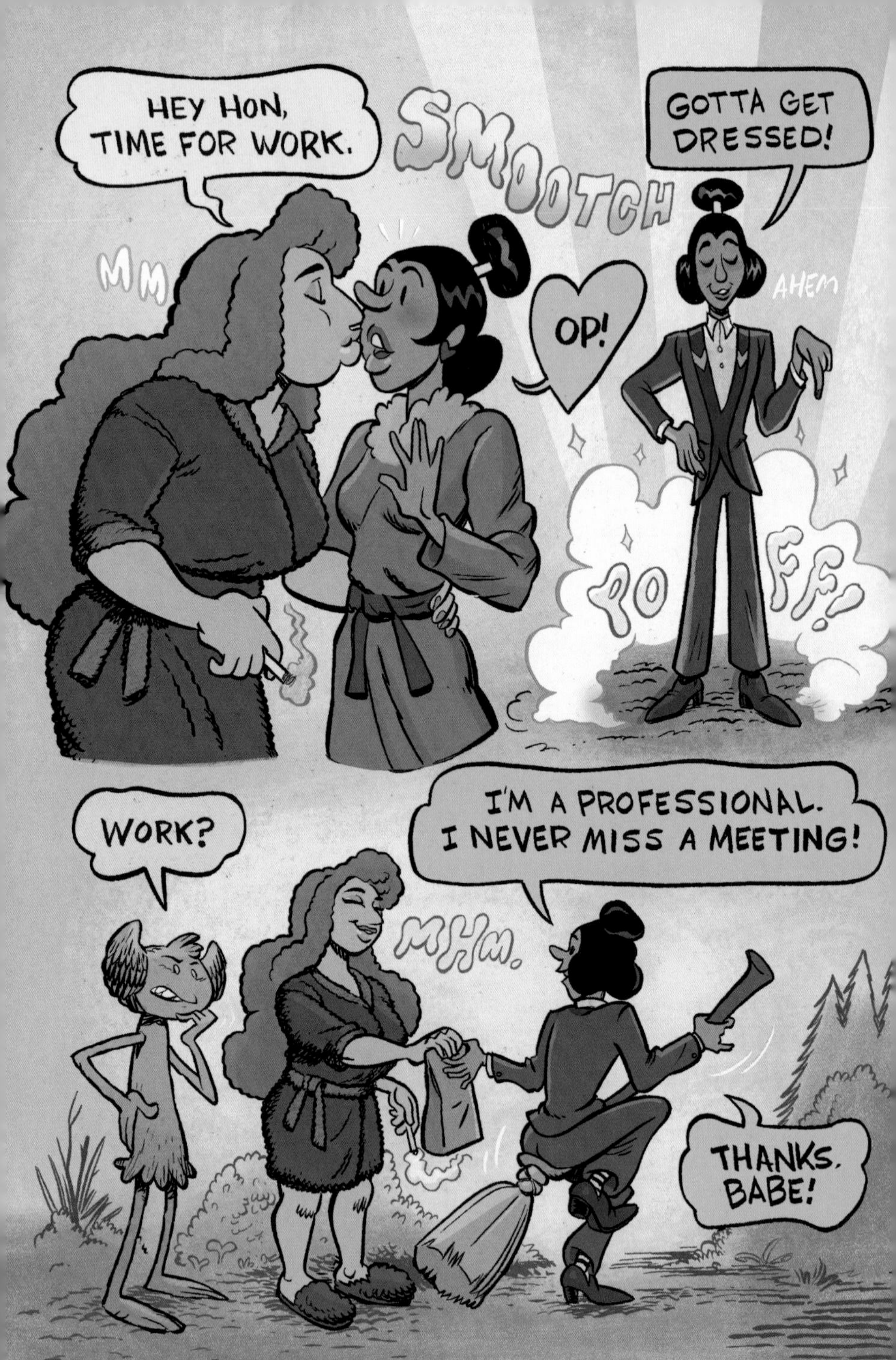
HEY HON, TIME FOR WORK.
SMOOTCH
GOTTA GET DRESSED!
MM
OP!
AHEM
POFF!
WORK?
I'M A PROFESSIONAL. I NEVER MISS A MEETING!
MHM.
THANKS, BABE!

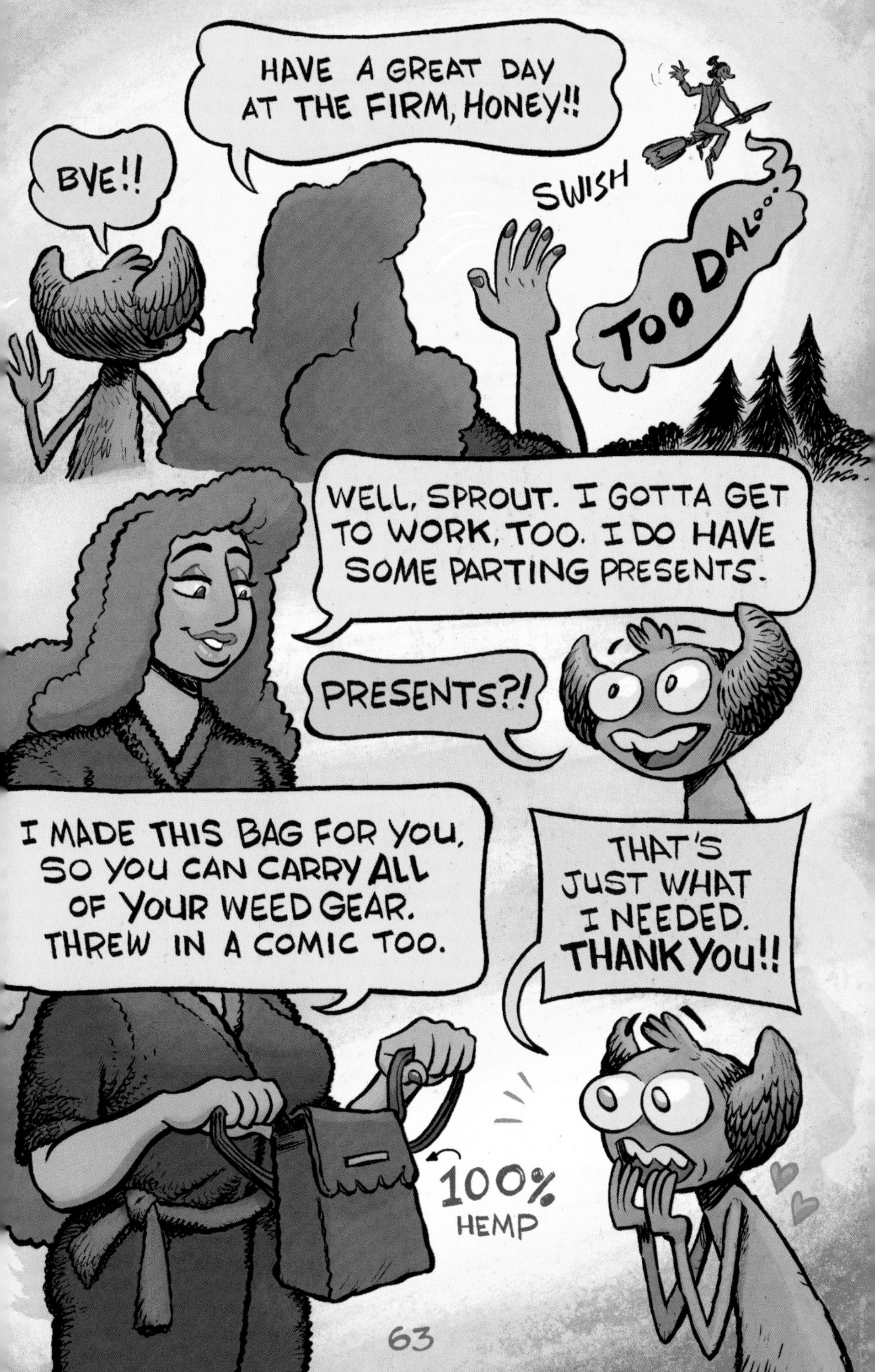
HAVE A GREAT DAY AT THE FIRM, HONEY!!
BYE!!
SWISH
TOO DALOOO
WELL, SPROUT. I GOTTA GET TO WORK, TOO. I DO HAVE SOME PARTING PRESENTS.
PRESENTS?!
I MADE THIS BAG FOR YOU, SO YOU CAN CARRY ALL OF YOUR WEED GEAR. THREW IN A COMIC TOO.
THAT'S JUST WHAT I NEEDED. THANK YOU!!
100% HEMP

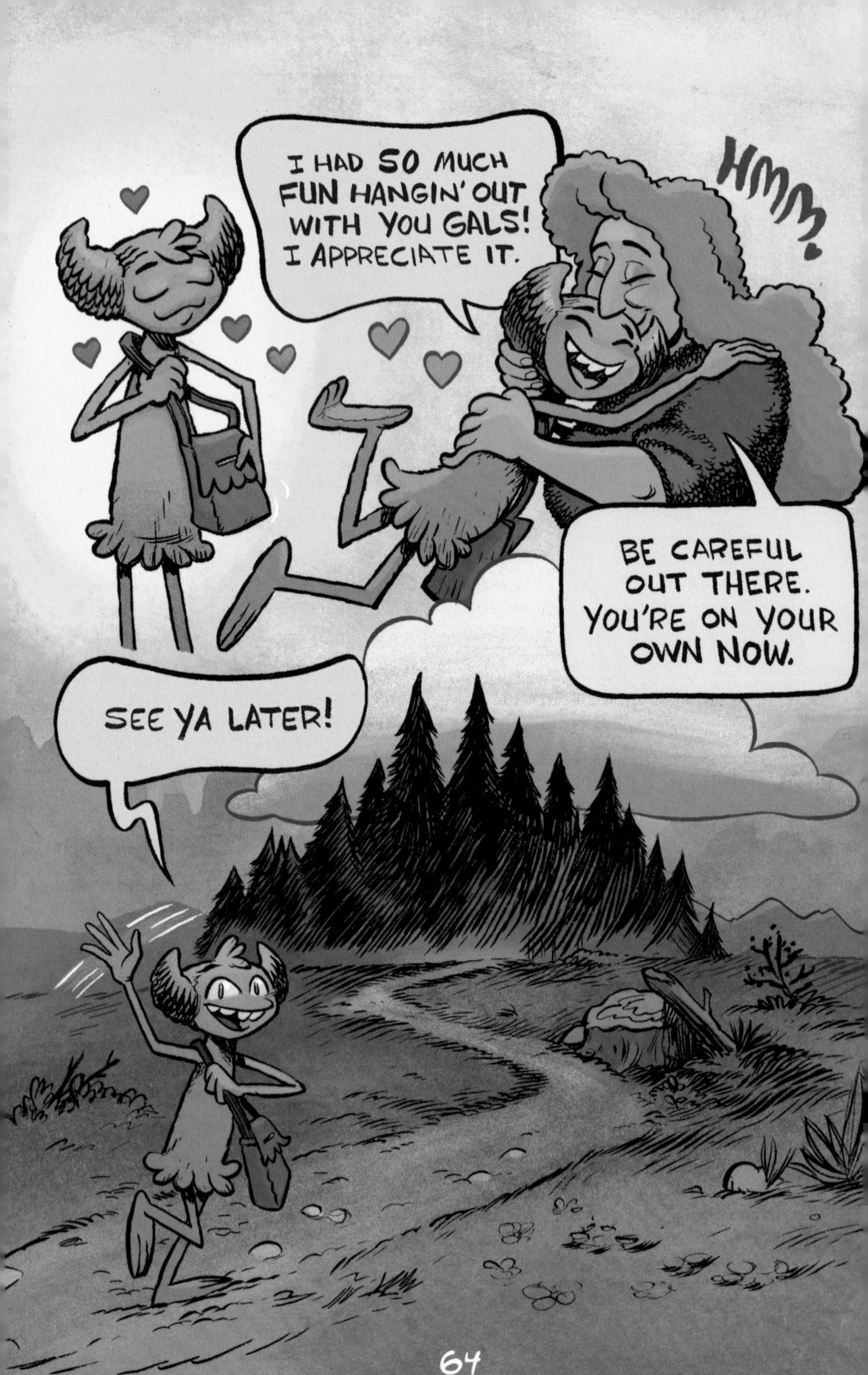
I HAD SO MUCH FUN HANGIN' OUT WITH YOU GALS! I APPRECIATE IT.
HMM
BE CAREFUL OUT THERE. YOU'RE ON YOUR OWN NOW.
SEE YA LATER!

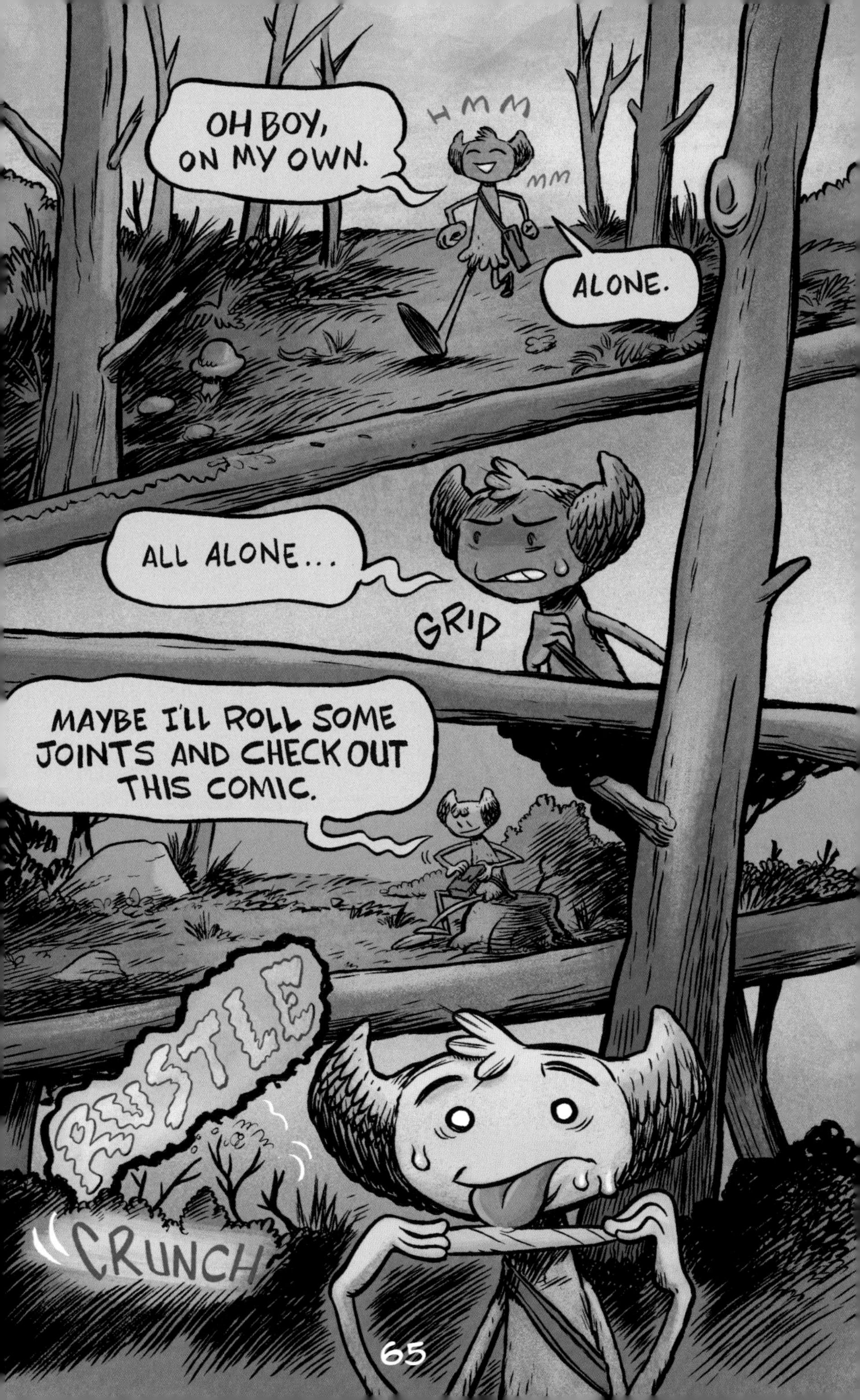
OH BOY, ON MY OWN.
HMM
MM
ALONE.
ALL ALONE...
GRIP
MAYBE I'LL ROLL SOME JOINTS AND CHECK OUT THIS COMIC.
RUSTLE
CRUNCH

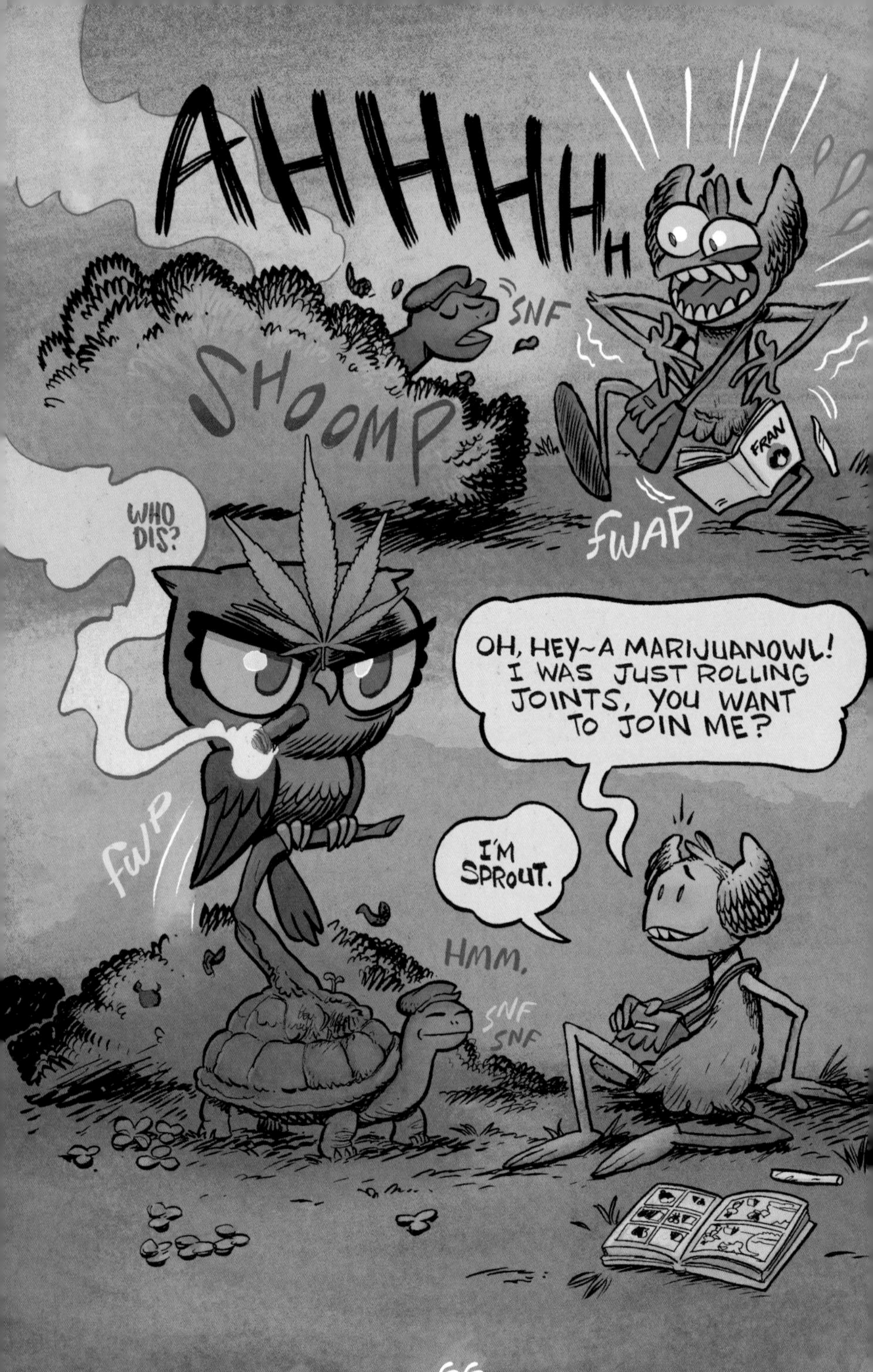
AHHHHH
SNF
SHOOMP
FRAN
FWAP
WHO DIS?
OH, HEY~A MARIJUANOWL! I WAS JUST ROLLING JOINTS, YOU WANT TO JOIN ME?
FWP
I'M SPROUT.
HMM.
SNF SNF

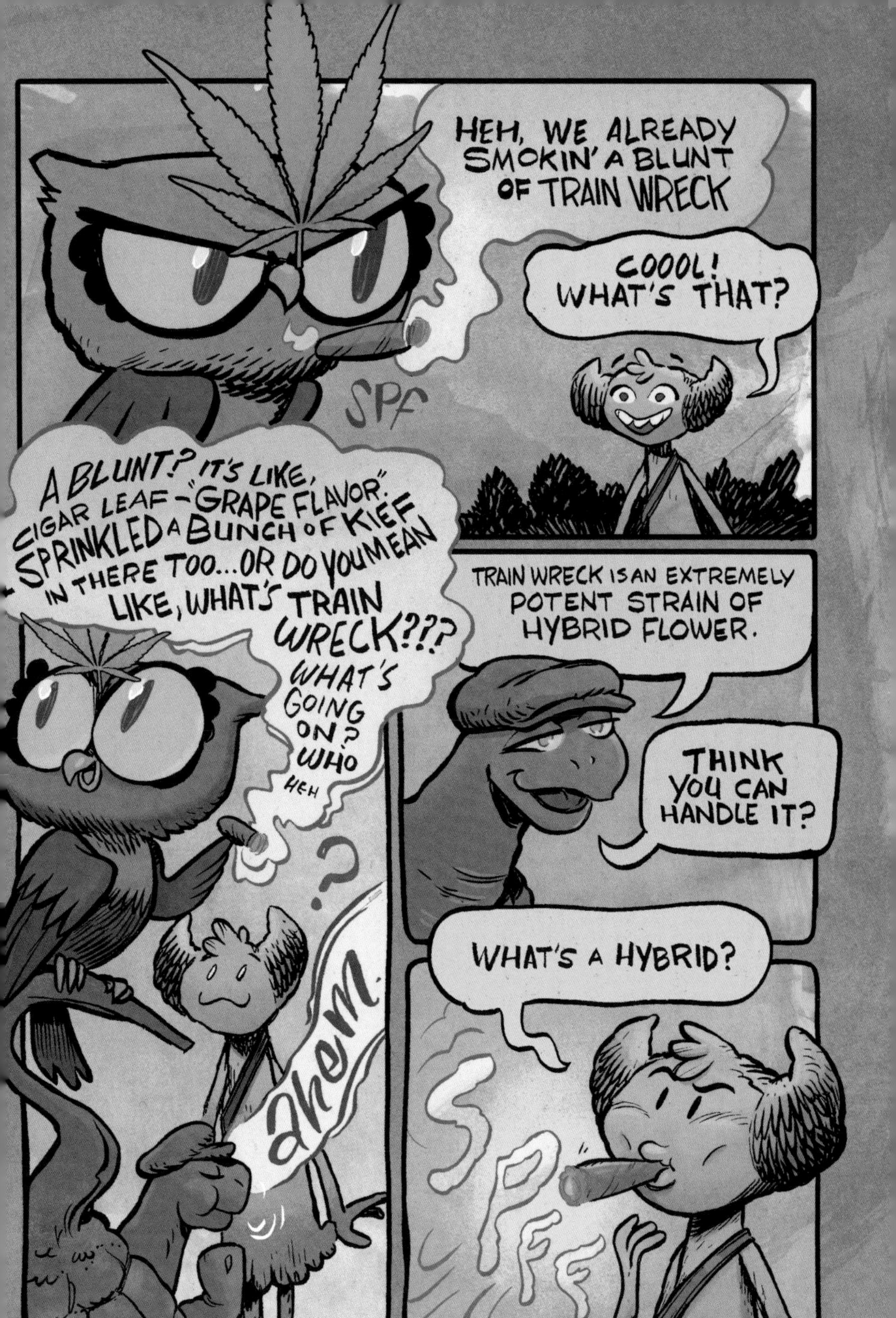
HEH, WE ALREADY SMOKIN' A BLUNT OF TRAIN WRECK
SPF
COOOL! WHAT'S THAT?
A BLUNT? IT'S LIKE, CIGAR LEAF - "GRAPE FLAVOR". SPRINKLED A BUNCH OF KIEF IN THERE TOO...OR DO YOU MEAN LIKE, WHAT'S TRAIN WRECK??? WHAT'S GOING ON? WHO HEH
TRAIN WRECK IS AN EXTREMELY POTENT STRAIN OF HYBRID FLOWER.
THINK YOU CAN HANDLE IT?
?
ahem.
WHAT'S A HYBRID?
SPFF

HYBRID

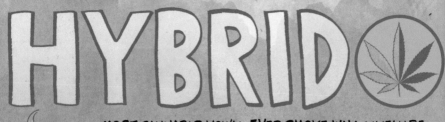

MOST CANNABIS YOU'LL **EVER** SMOKE WILL LIKELY BE SOME KIND OF HYBRID. GROWERS CROSS **STRAINS** TO GET TRAITS SUCH AS HIGH **THC** CONTENT, ***SCENTS, FLAVORS,*** OR EVEN JUST TO **SEE** *WHAT HAPPENS!*

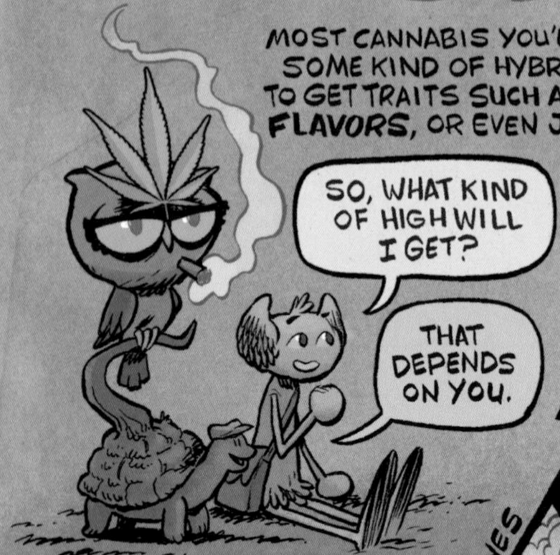
SO, WHAT KIND OF HIGH WILL I GET?
THAT DEPENDS ON YOU.

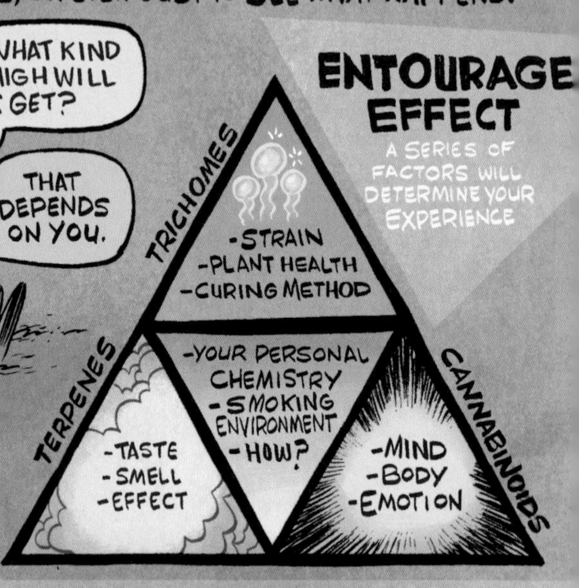
ENTOURAGE EFFECT
A SERIES OF FACTORS WILL DETERMINE YOUR EXPERIENCE
TRICHOMES
-STRAIN
-PLANT HEALTH
-CURING METHOD
TERPENES
-TASTE
-SMELL
-EFFECT
-YOUR PERSONAL CHEMISTRY
-SMOKING ENVIRONMENT
-HOW?
CANNABINOIDS
-MIND
-BODY
-EMOTION

HYBRIDS CAN BE BRED FOR A ***SATIVA-TYPE*** MENTAL HIGH BUT WITH THE ***FLOWERING*** TIMES OF AN **INDICA**.

EVERYONE IS AFFECTED DIFFERENTLY!

THERE MAY EVEN BE A STRAIN OUT THERE ***PERFECTLY*** SUITED TO YOU. EXPERT GROWERS ARE ALWAYS LOOKING FOR UNIQUE COMBINATIONS.

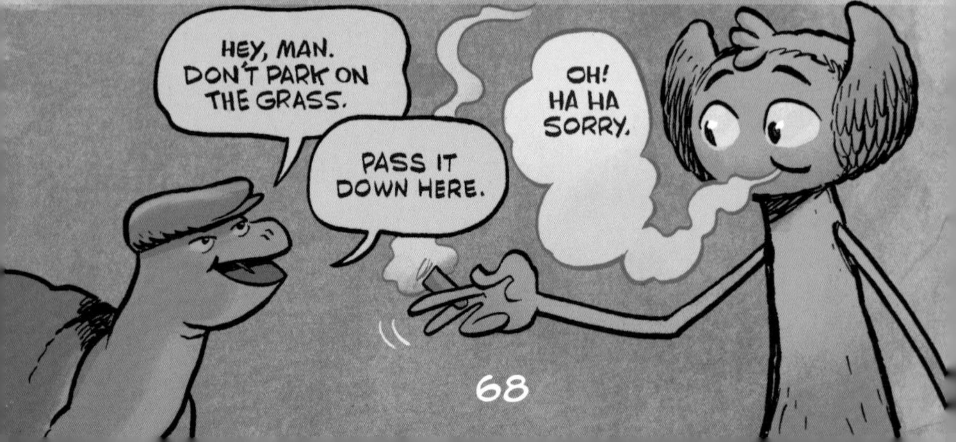
HEY, MAN. DON'T PARK ON THE GRASS.
PASS IT DOWN HERE.
OH! HA HA SORRY.

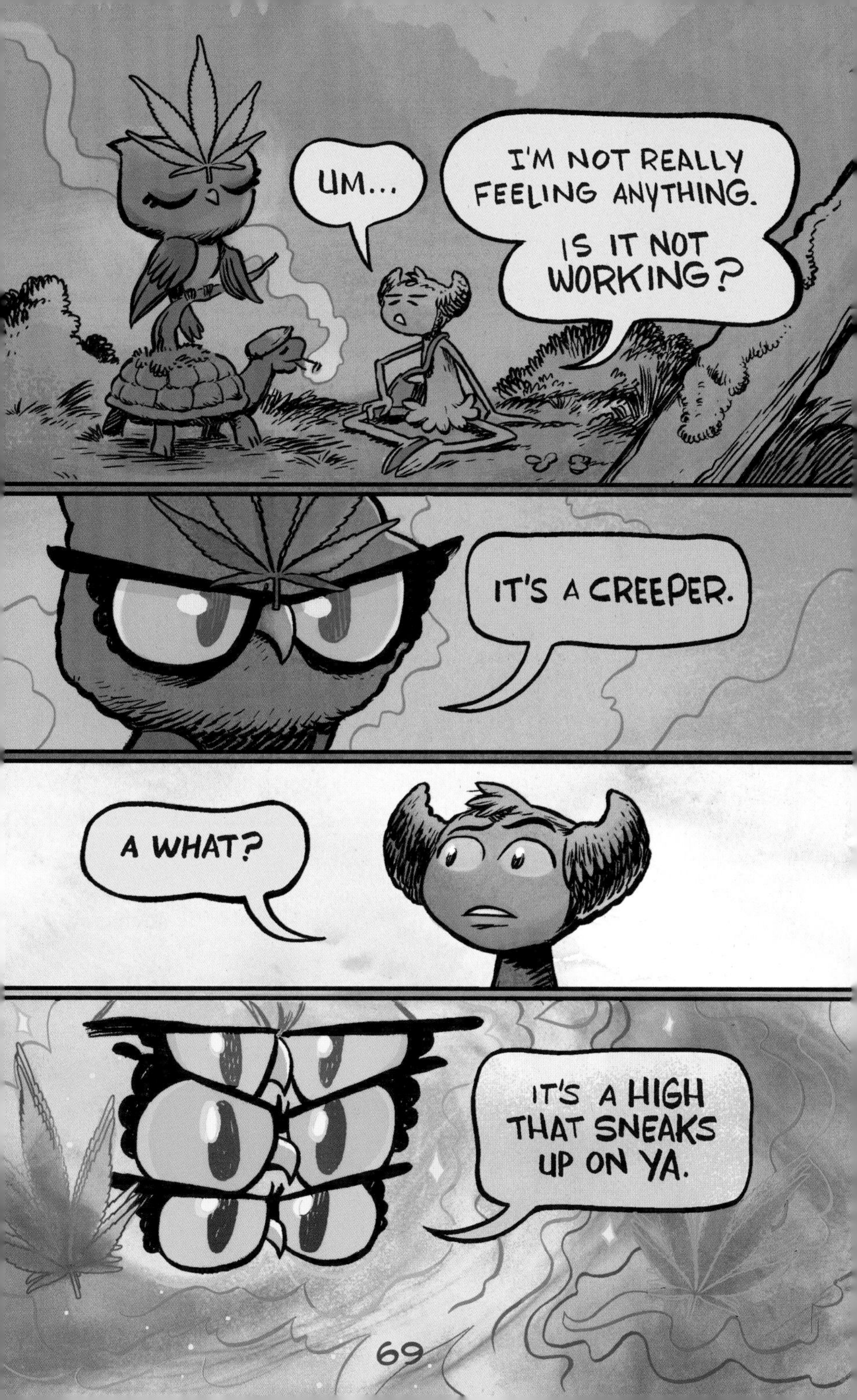
UM...
I'M NOT REALLY FEELING ANYTHING.
IS IT NOT WORKING?
IT'S A CREEPER.
A WHAT?
IT'S A HIGH THAT SNEAKS UP ON YA.

SIGNS THAT YOU MAY BE OVER-BAKED, GREENING OUT, WICKED STONED, ROYALLY BLAZED, OR JUST...

TOO HIGH

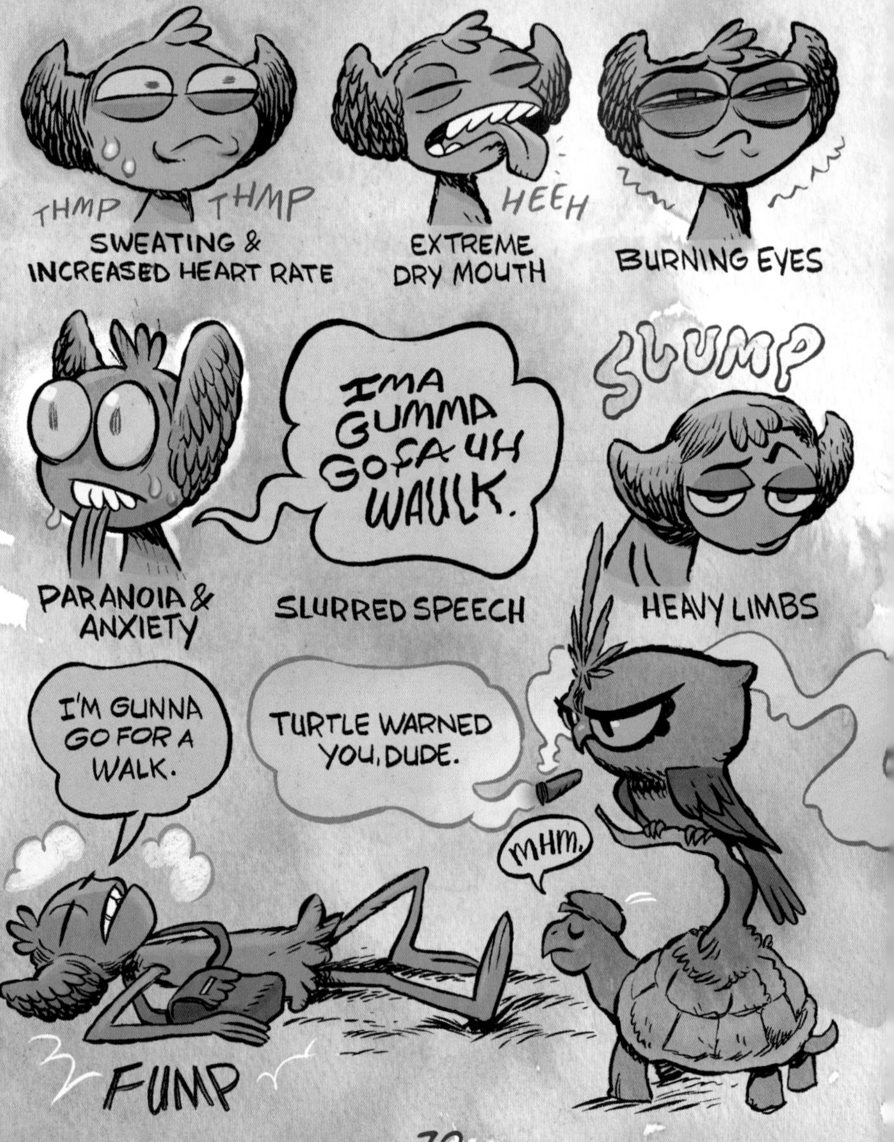
THMP THMP
SWEATING & INCREASED HEART RATE
HEEEH
EXTREME DRY MOUTH
BURNING EYES
IMA GUMMA GOFA UH WAULK.
SLUMP
PARANOIA & ANXIETY
SLURRED SPEECH
HEAVY LIMBS
I'M GUNNA GO FOR A WALK.
TURTLE WARNED YOU, DUDE.
MHM.
FUMP

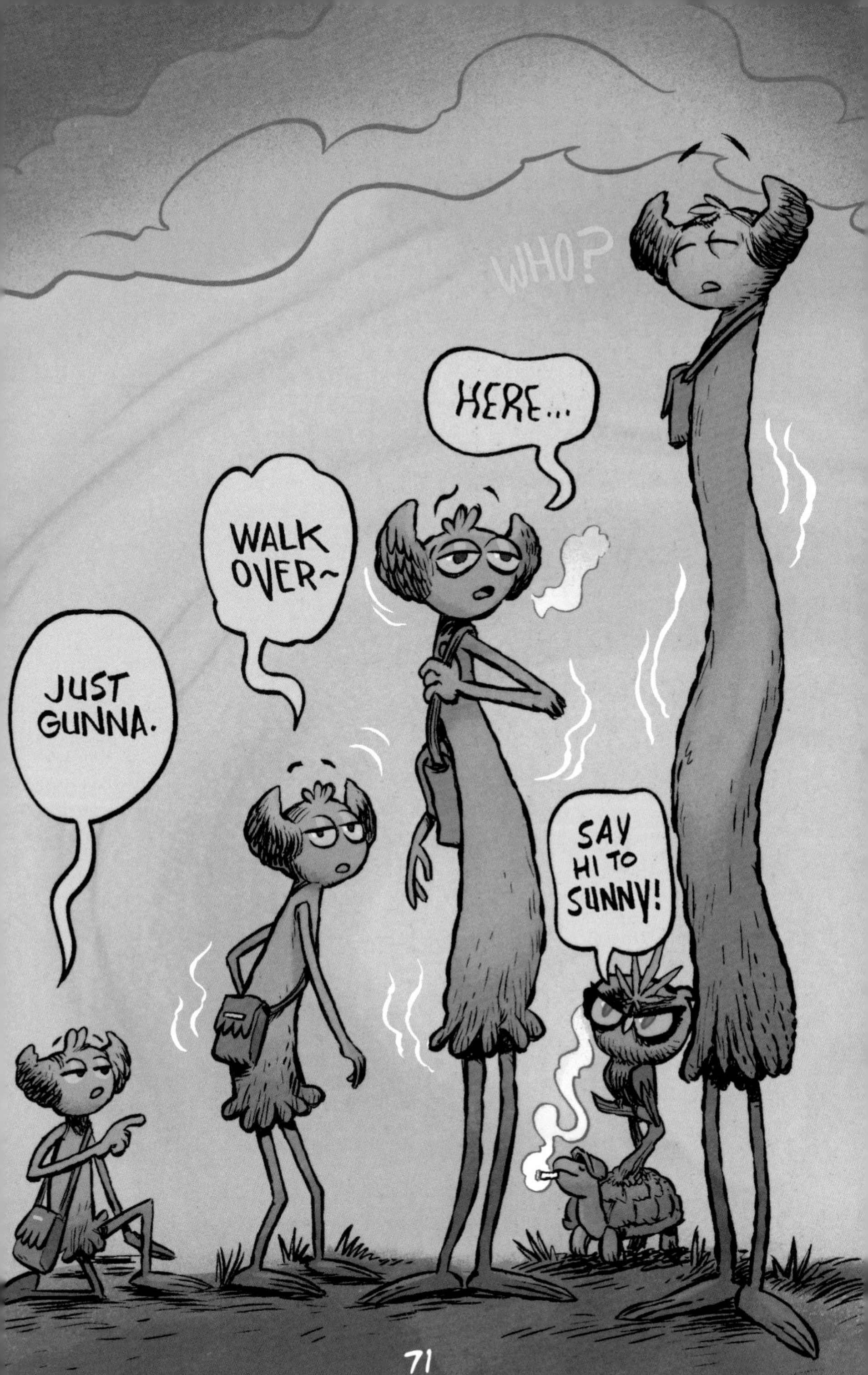
JUST GUNNA.
WALK OVER~
HERE...
WHO?
SAY HI TO SUNNY!

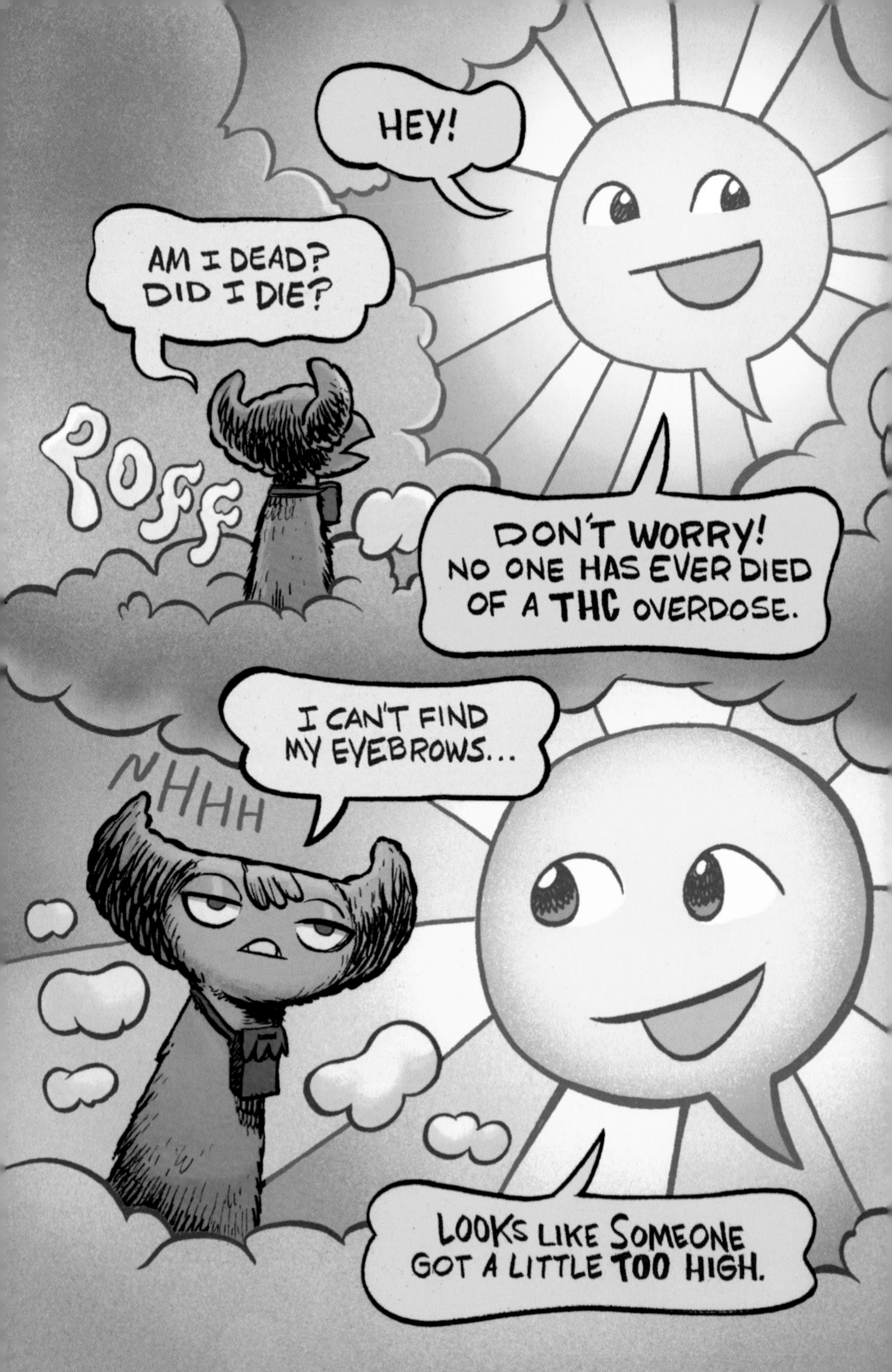
HEY!
AM I DEAD? DID I DIE?
POFF
DON'T WORRY! NO ONE HAS EVER DIED OF A THC OVERDOSE.
I CAN'T FIND MY EYEBROWS...
NHHH
LOOKS LIKE SOMEONE GOT A LITTLE TOO HIGH.

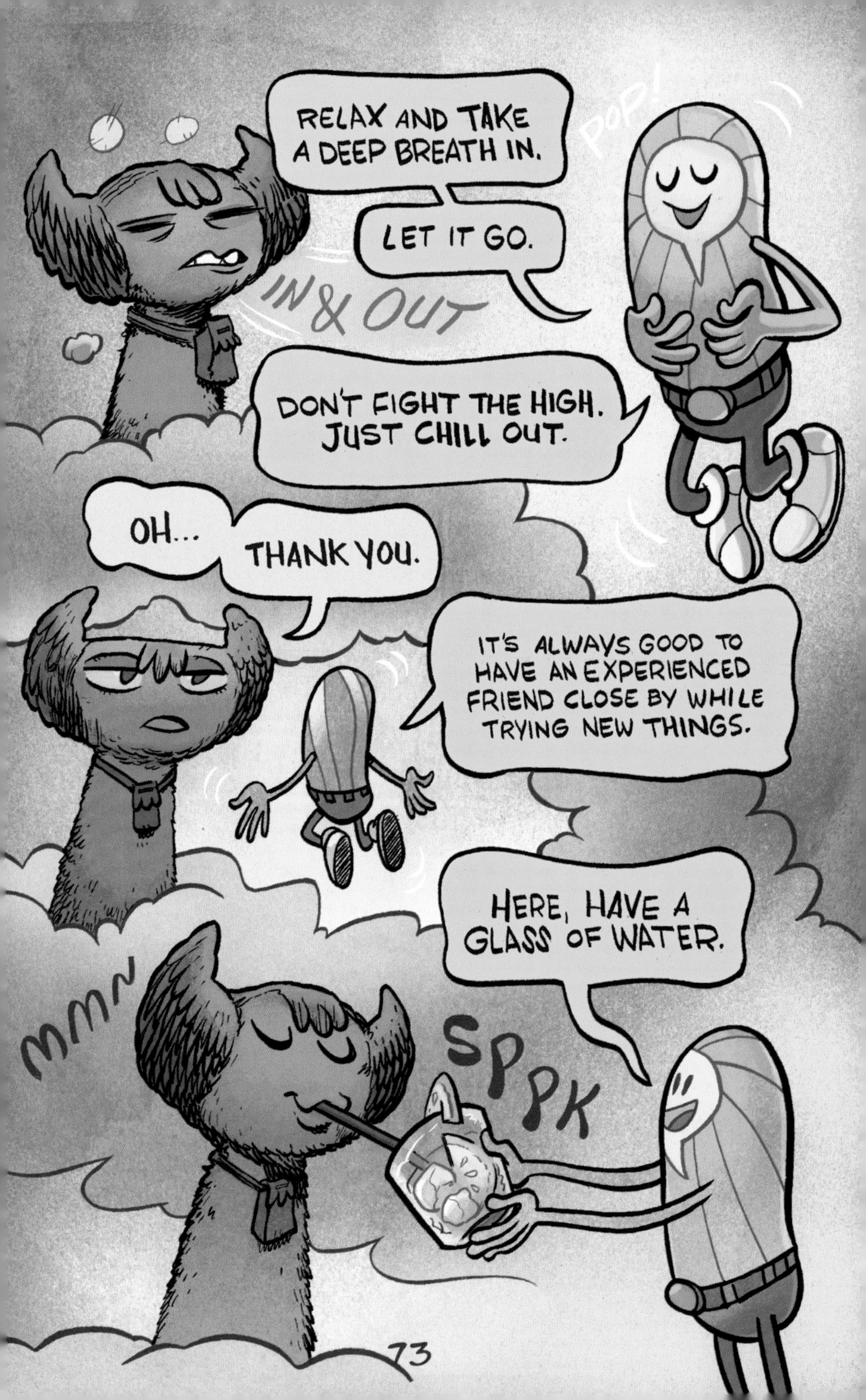
RELAX AND TAKE A DEEP BREATH IN.
POP!
LET IT GO.
IN & OUT
DON'T FIGHT THE HIGH. JUST CHILL OUT.
OH...
THANK YOU.
IT'S ALWAYS GOOD TO HAVE AN EXPERIENCED FRIEND CLOSE BY WHILE TRYING NEW THINGS.
HERE, HAVE A GLASS OF WATER.
MMM
SPPK

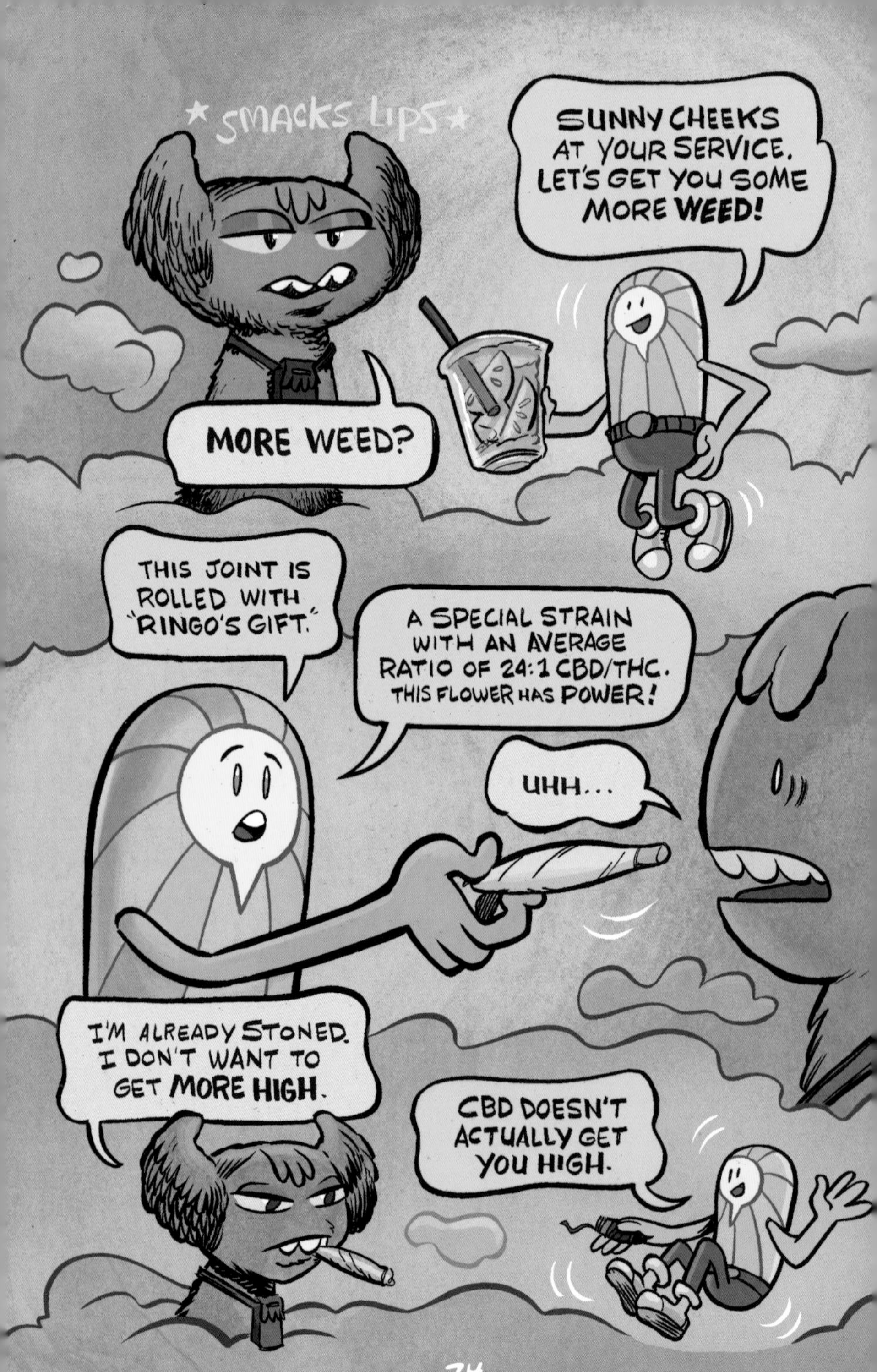

★SMACKS LIPS★
SUNNY CHEEKS AT YOUR SERVICE. LET'S GET YOU SOME MORE WEED!
MORE WEED?
THIS JOINT IS ROLLED WITH "RINGO'S GIFT."
A SPECIAL STRAIN WITH AN AVERAGE RATIO OF 24:1 CBD/THC. THIS FLOWER HAS POWER!
UHH...
I'M ALREADY STONED. I DON'T WANT TO GET MORE HIGH.
CBD DOESN'T ACTUALLY GET YOU HIGH.

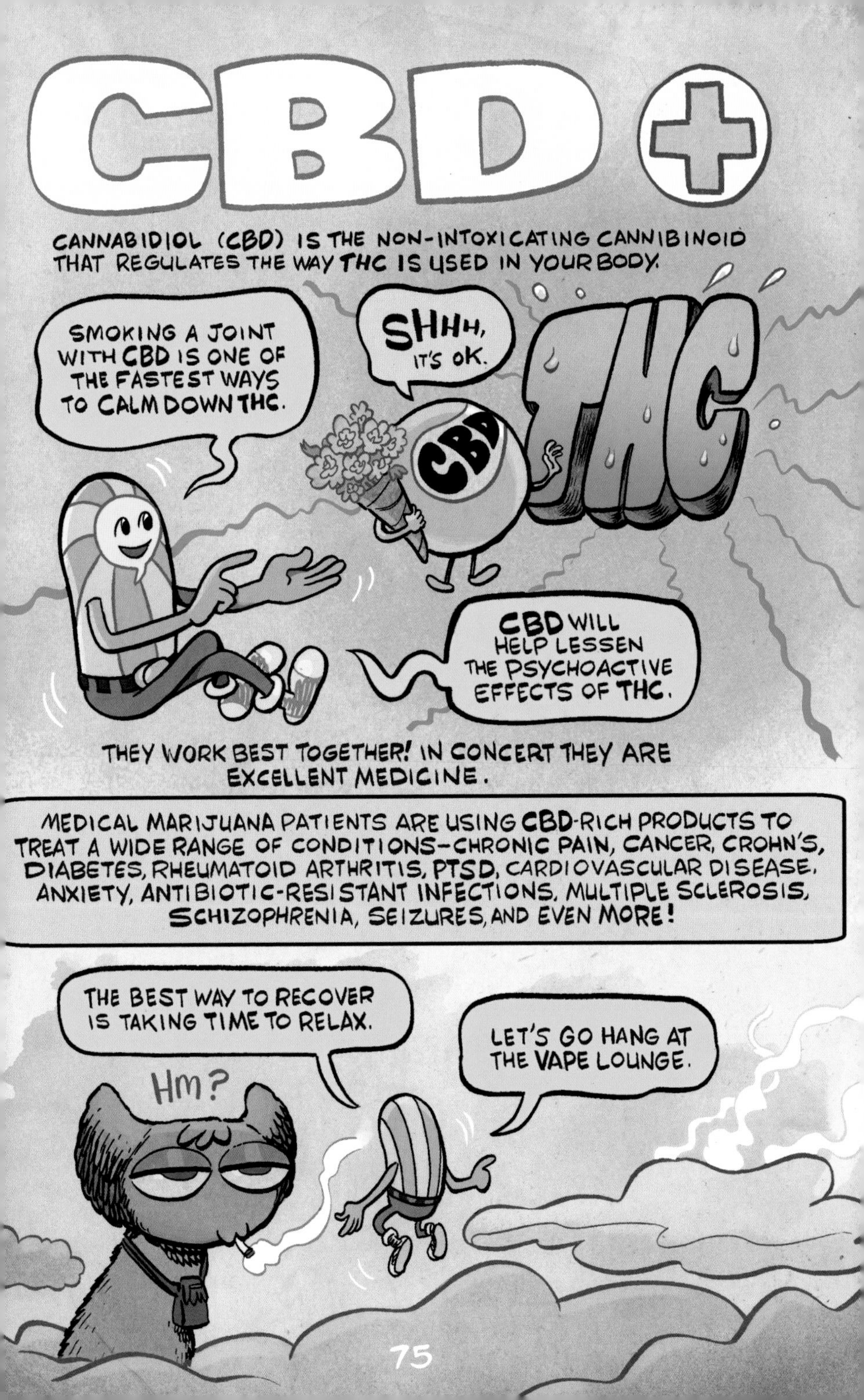
CBD
CANNABIDIOL (CBD) IS THE NON-INTOXICATING CANNIBINOID THAT REGULATES THE WAY THC IS USED IN YOUR BODY.
SMOKING A JOINT WITH CBD IS ONE OF THE FASTEST WAYS TO CALM DOWN THC.
SHHH, IT'S OK.
CBD
THC
CBD WILL HELP LESSEN THE PSYCHOACTIVE EFFECTS OF THC.
THEY WORK BEST TOGETHER! IN CONCERT THEY ARE EXCELLENT MEDICINE.
MEDICAL MARIJUANA PATIENTS ARE USING CBD-RICH PRODUCTS TO TREAT A WIDE RANGE OF CONDITIONS—CHRONIC PAIN, CANCER, CROHN'S, DIABETES, RHEUMATOID ARTHRITIS, PTSD, CARDIOVASCULAR DISEASE, ANXIETY, ANTIBIOTIC-RESISTANT INFECTIONS, MULTIPLE SCLEROSIS, SCHIZOPHRENIA, SEIZURES, AND EVEN MORE!
THE BEST WAY TO RECOVER IS TAKING TIME TO RELAX.
Hm?
LET'S GO HANG AT THE VAPE LOUNGE.

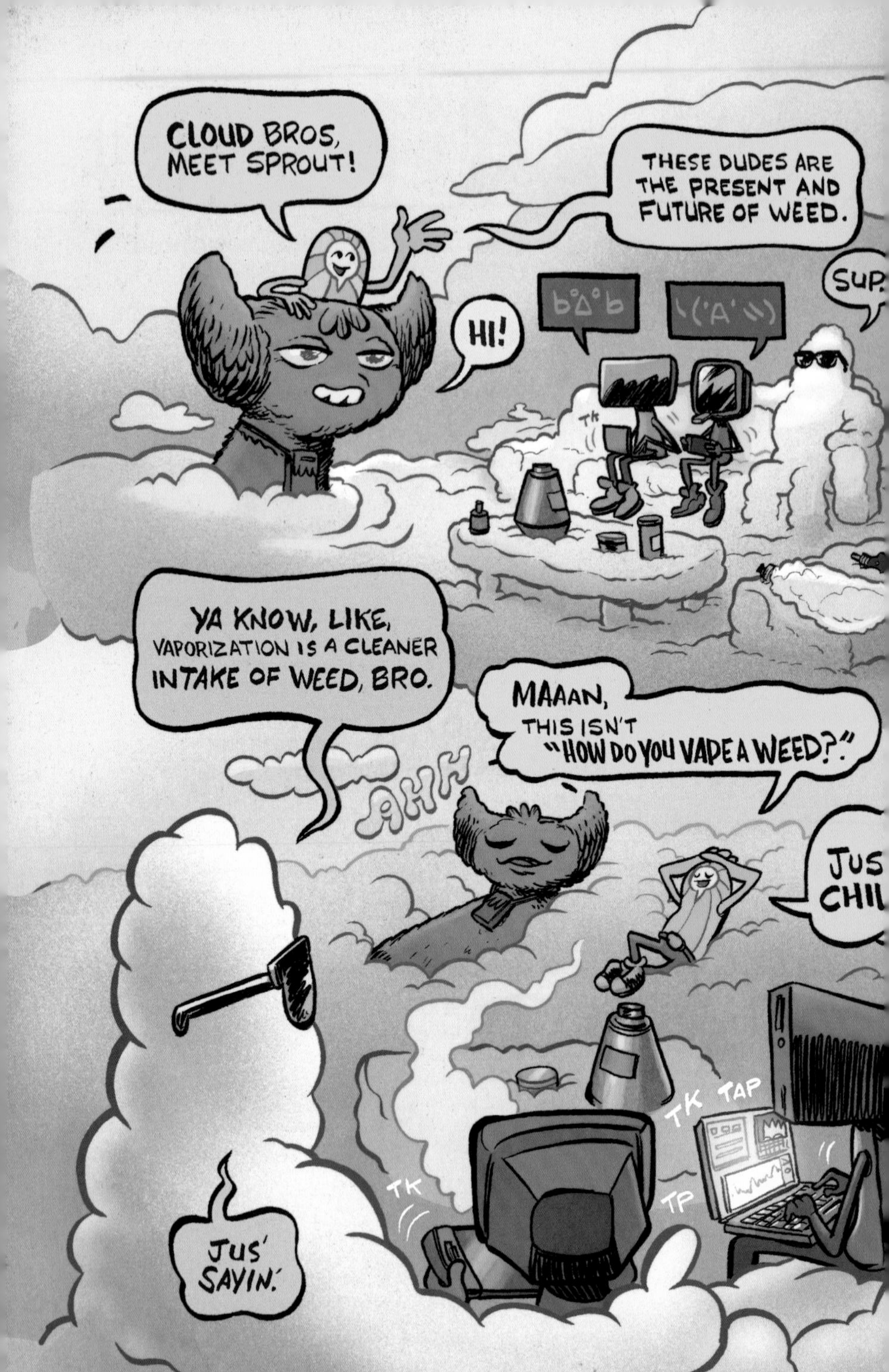

CLOUD BROS, MEET SPROUT!
THESE DUDES ARE THE PRESENT AND FUTURE OF WEED.
HI!
SUP.
YA KNOW, LIKE, VAPORIZATION IS A CLEANER INTAKE OF WEED, BRO.
MAAAN, THIS ISN'T "HOW DO YOU VAPE A WEED?"
AHH
JUS' SAYIN.'
TK TAP
TK
TP

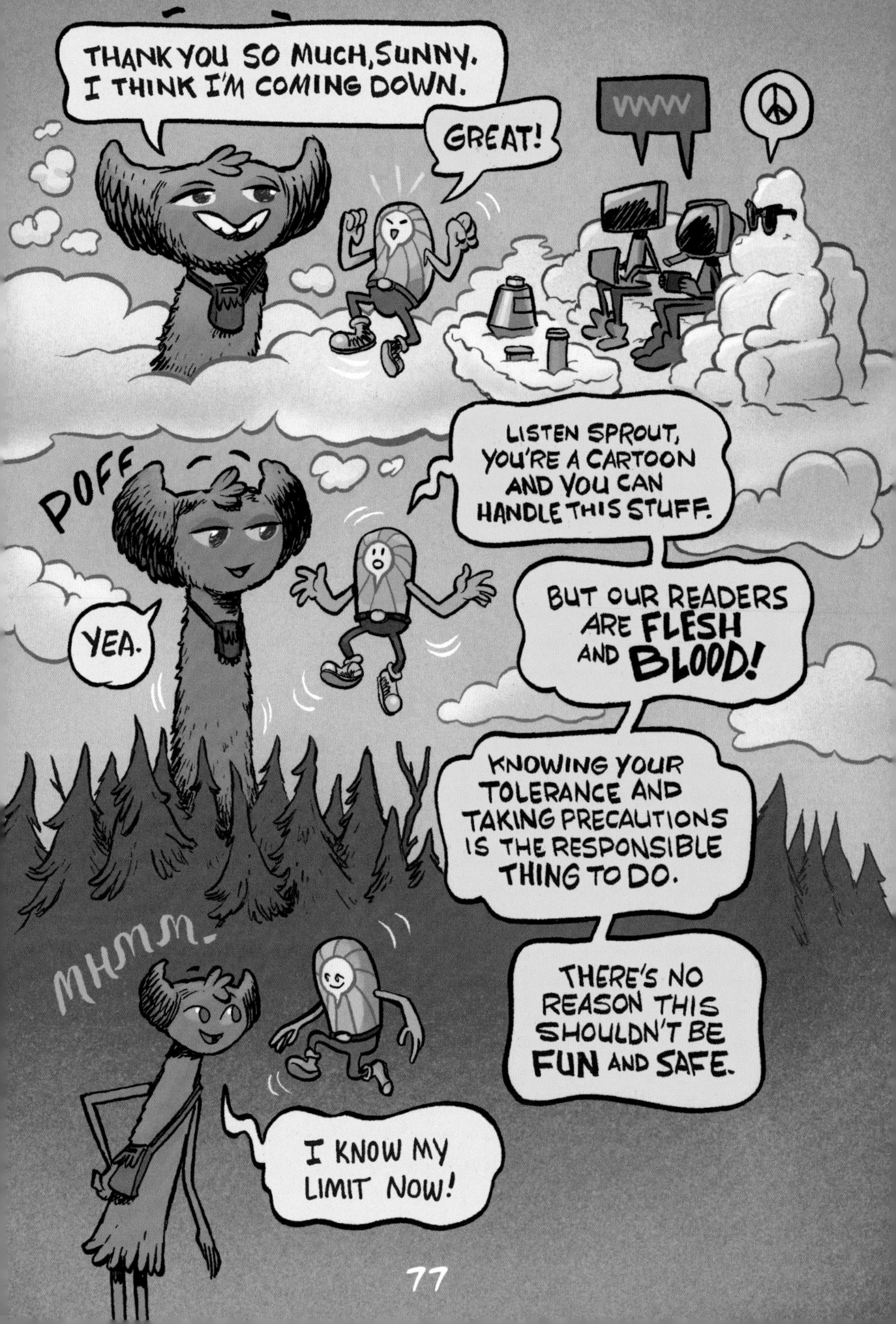
THANK YOU SO MUCH, SUNNY. I THINK I'M COMING DOWN.
GREAT!
LISTEN SPROUT, YOU'RE A CARTOON AND YOU CAN HANDLE THIS STUFF.
POFF
YEA.
BUT OUR READERS ARE FLESH AND BLOOD!
KNOWING YOUR TOLERANCE AND TAKING PRECAUTIONS IS THE RESPONSIBLE THING TO DO.
MHMM.
THERE'S NO REASON THIS SHOULDN'T BE FUN AND SAFE.
I KNOW MY LIMIT NOW!

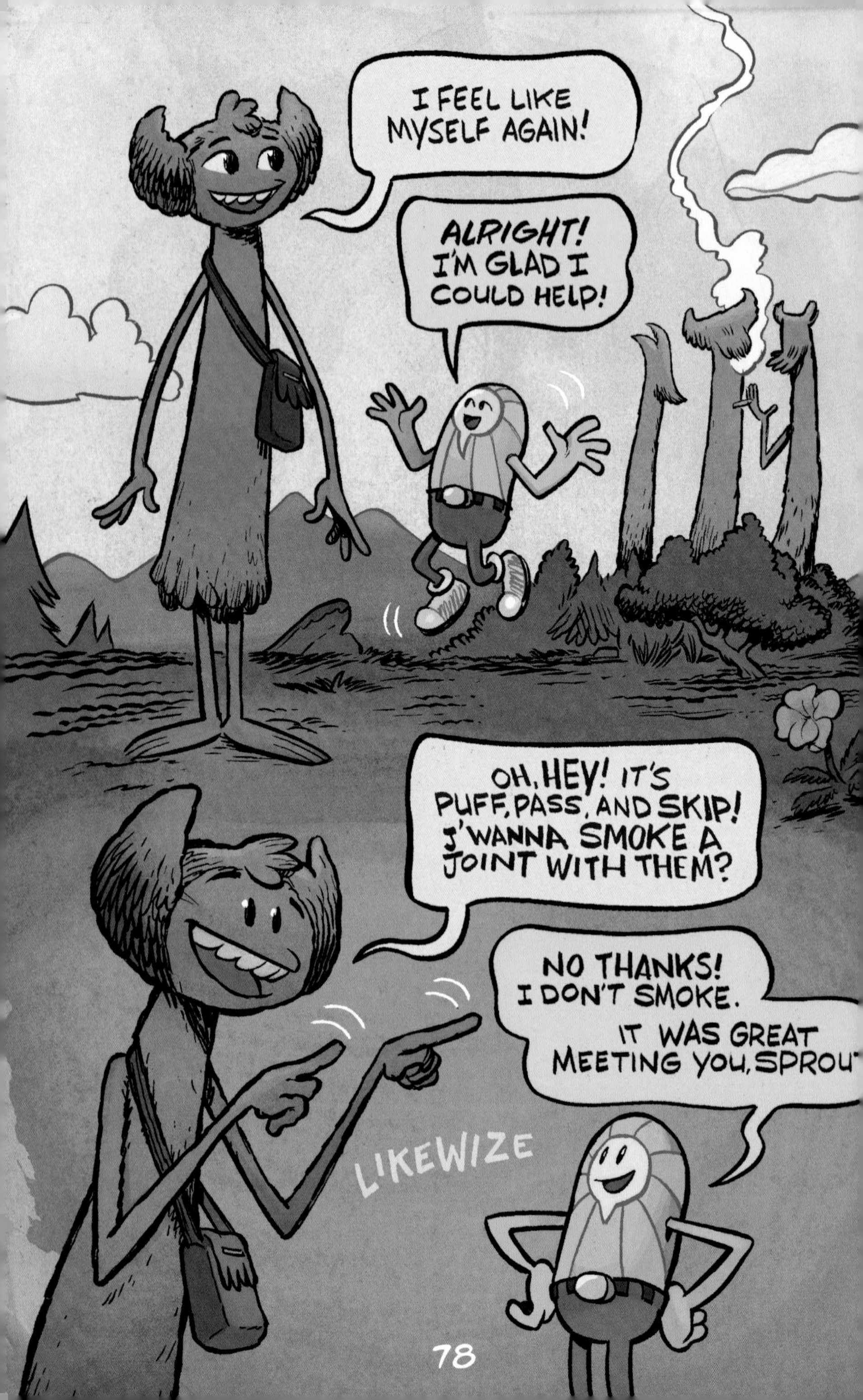
I FEEL LIKE MYSELF AGAIN!
ALRIGHT! I'M GLAD I COULD HELP!
OH, HEY! IT'S PUFF, PASS, AND SKIP! J'WANNA SMOKE A JOINT WITH THEM?
NO THANKS! I DON'T SMOKE.
IT WAS GREAT MEETING YOU, SPROU
LIKEWIZE

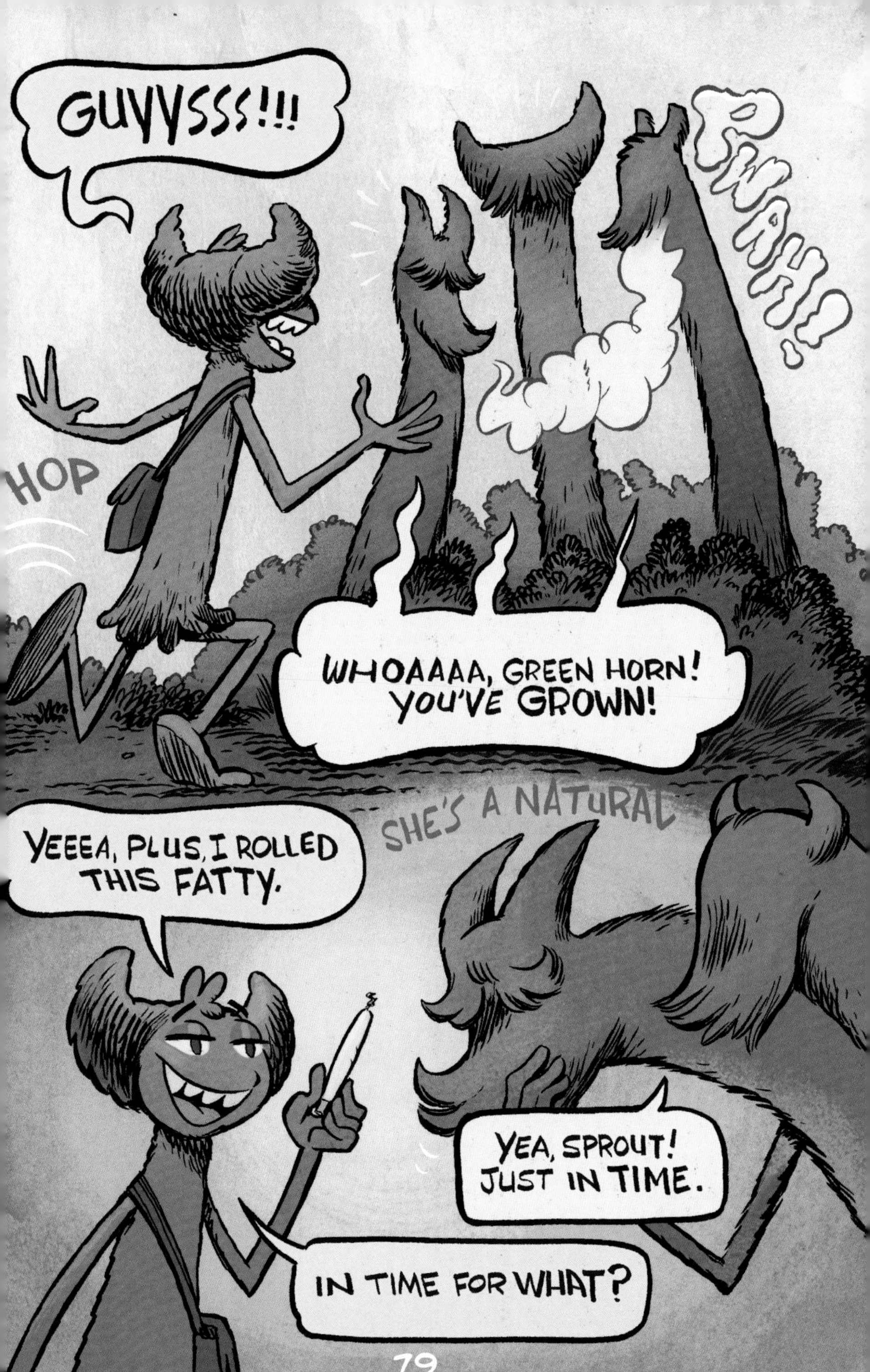
GUYYSSSS!!!
PWAH!!
HOP
WHOAAAA, GREEN HORN! YOU'VE GROWN!
SHE'S A NATURAL
YEEEA, PLUS, I ROLLED THIS FATTY.
YEA, SPROUT! JUST IN TIME.
IN TIME FOR WHAT?

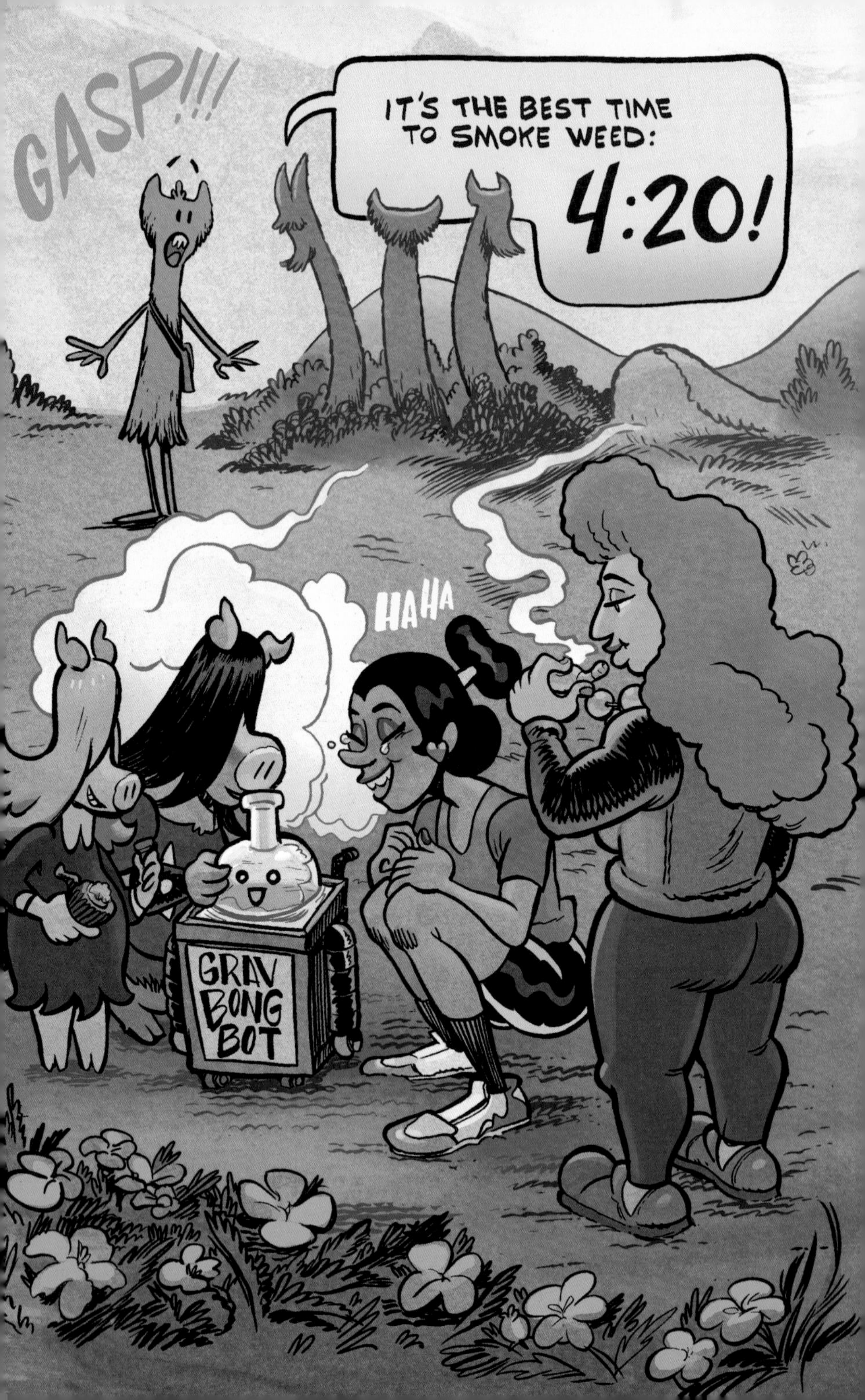
GASP!!!
IT'S THE BEST TIME
TO SMOKE WEED:
4:20!
HAHA
GRAV
BONG
BOT

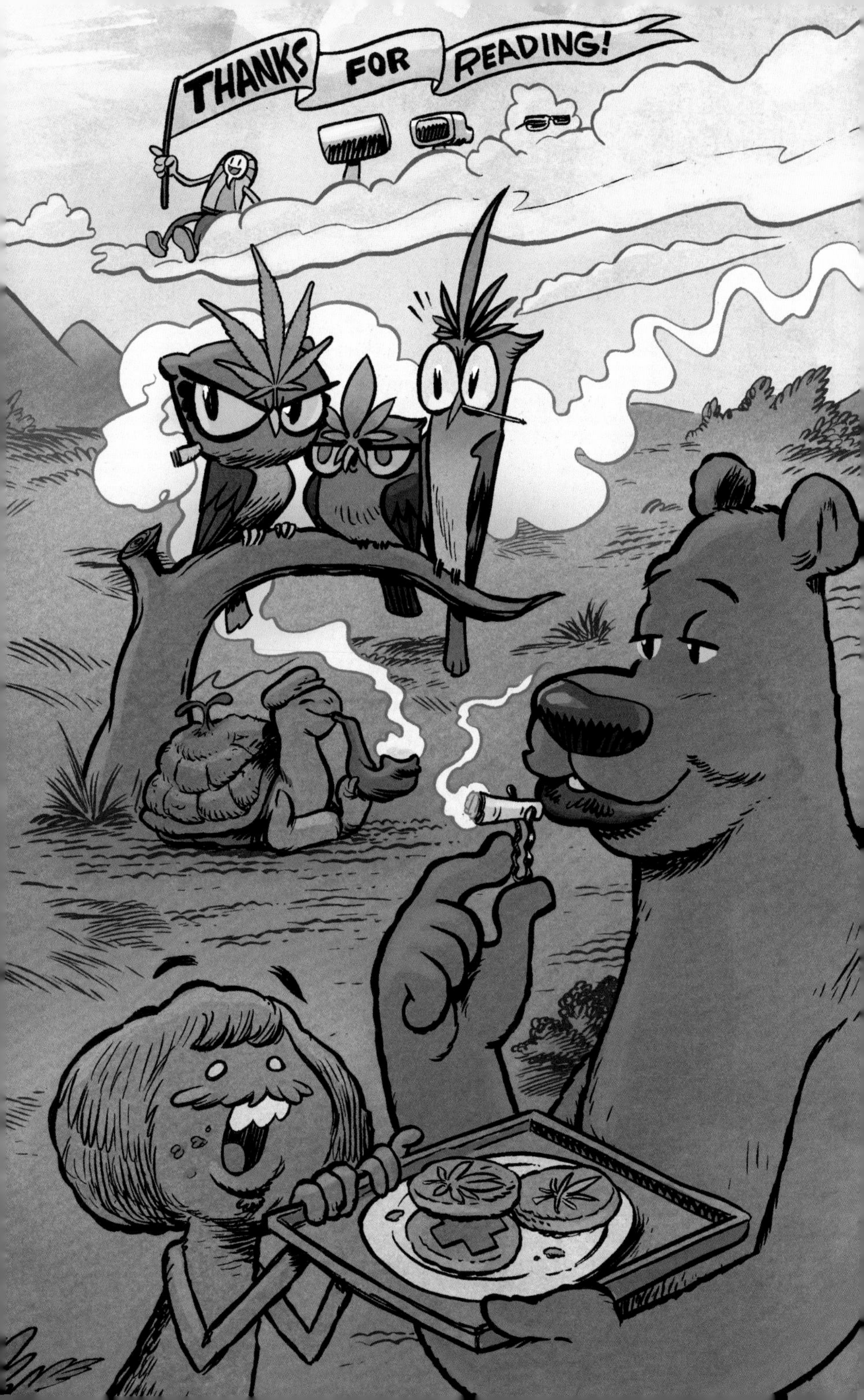
THANKS FOR READING!

FINAL THOUGHTS:

SMOKING CAN BE HABIT FORMING. PAY ATTENTION TO YOUR CONSUMPTION. HAVE RESPECT FOR THIS BEAUTIFUL, POWERFUL, AND POTENT PLANT!

ASK YOURSELF: HOW DO *YOU* LIKE TO SMOKE A WEED?

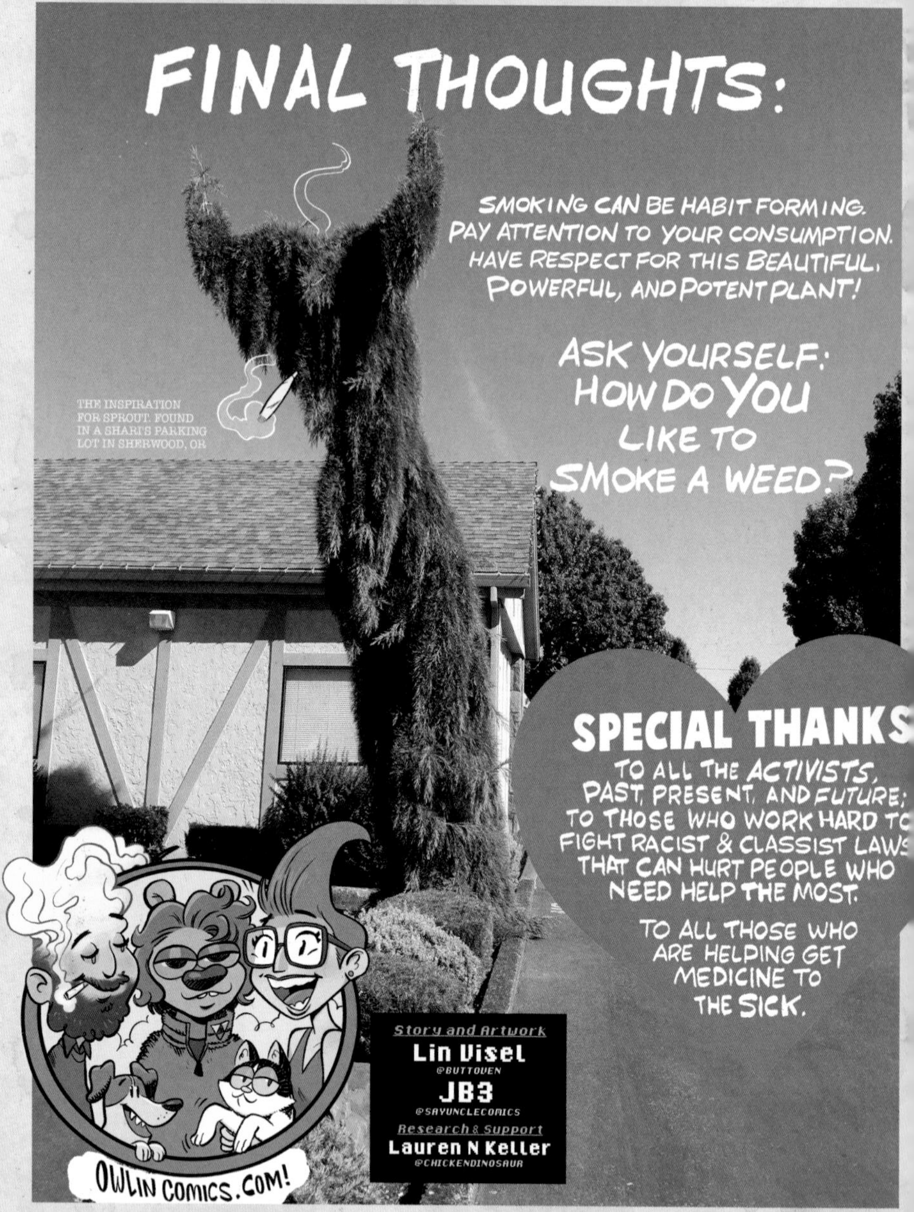
THE INSPIRATION FOR SPROUT. FOUND IN A SHARI'S PARKING LOT IN SHERWOOD, OR
OWLIN COMICS.COM!

SPECIAL THANKS

TO ALL THE *ACTIVISTS*, PAST, PRESENT, AND *FUTURE*; TO THOSE WHO WORK HARD TO FIGHT RACIST & CLASSIST LAWS THAT CAN HURT PEOPLE WHO NEED HELP THE MOST.

TO ALL THOSE WHO ARE HELPING GET MEDICINE TO THE SICK.

Story and Artwork
Lin Visel
@BUTTOVEN
JB3
@SAYUNCLECOMICS
Research & Support
Lauren N Keller
@CHICKENDINOSAUR

THANK YOU

TO THE FOLLOWING RESOURCES:

THE SCIENCE OF MARIJUANA BY LESLIE L. IVERSEN

WEED: THE USER'S GUIDE BY DAVID SCHMADER

THE POT BOOK: A COMPLETE GUIDE TO CANNABIS **EDITED BY JULIE HOLLAND M.D.**

LEAFLY.COM NORML.ORG PROJECTCBD.ORG

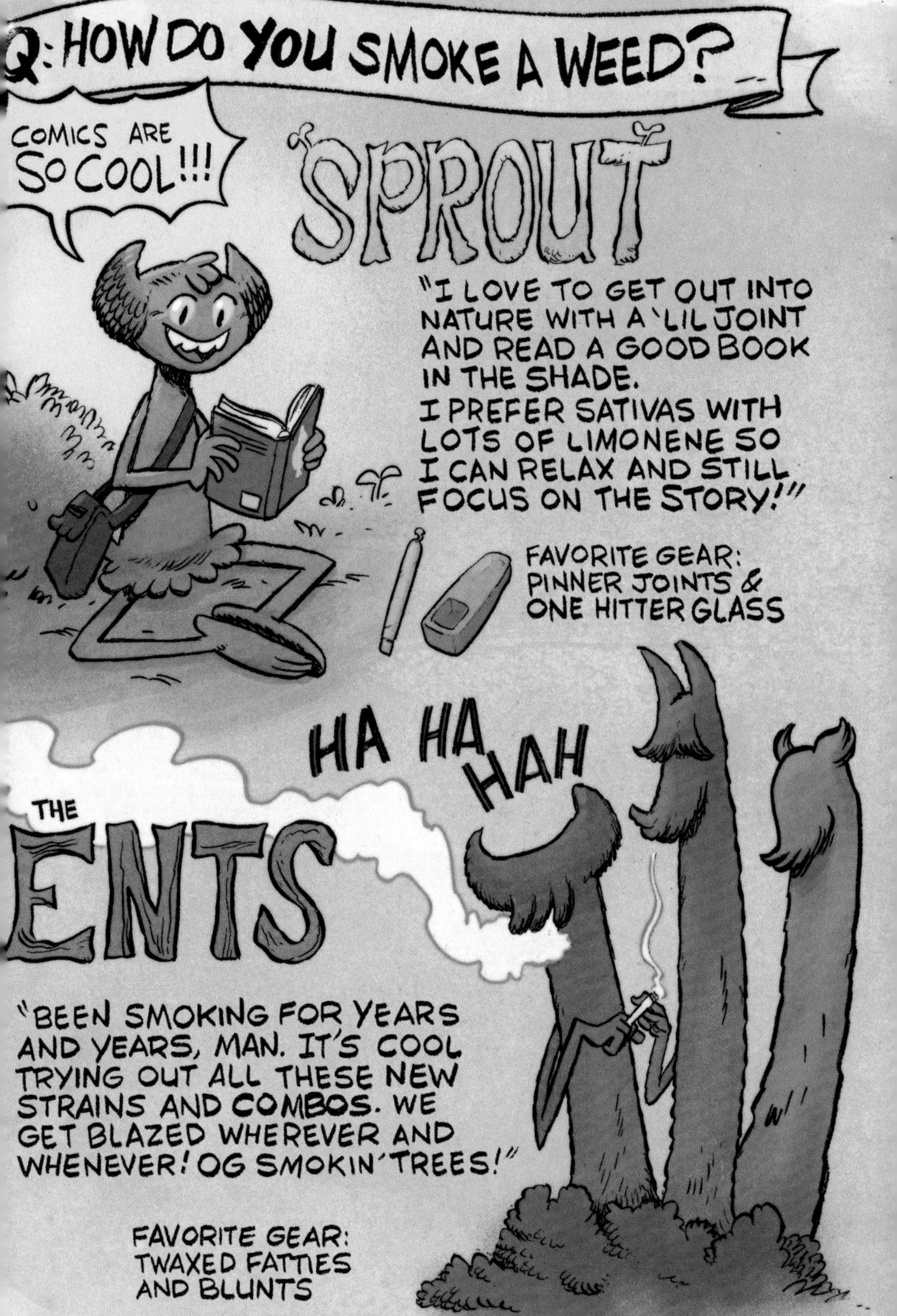
Q: HOW DO YOU SMOKE A WEED?
COMICS ARE SO COOL!!!
SPROUT
"I LOVE TO GET OUT INTO NATURE WITH A 'LIL JOINT AND READ A GOOD BOOK IN THE SHADE.
I PREFER SATIVAS WITH LOTS OF LIMONENE SO I CAN RELAX AND STILL FOCUS ON THE STORY!"
FAVORITE GEAR: PINNER JOINTS & ONE HITTER GLASS
HA HA HAH
THE ENTS
"BEEN SMOKING FOR YEARS AND YEARS, MAN. IT'S COOL TRYING OUT ALL THESE NEW STRAINS AND COMBOS. WE GET BLAZED WHEREVER AND WHENEVER! OG SMOKIN' TREES!"
FAVORITE GEAR: TWAXED FATTIES AND BLUNTS

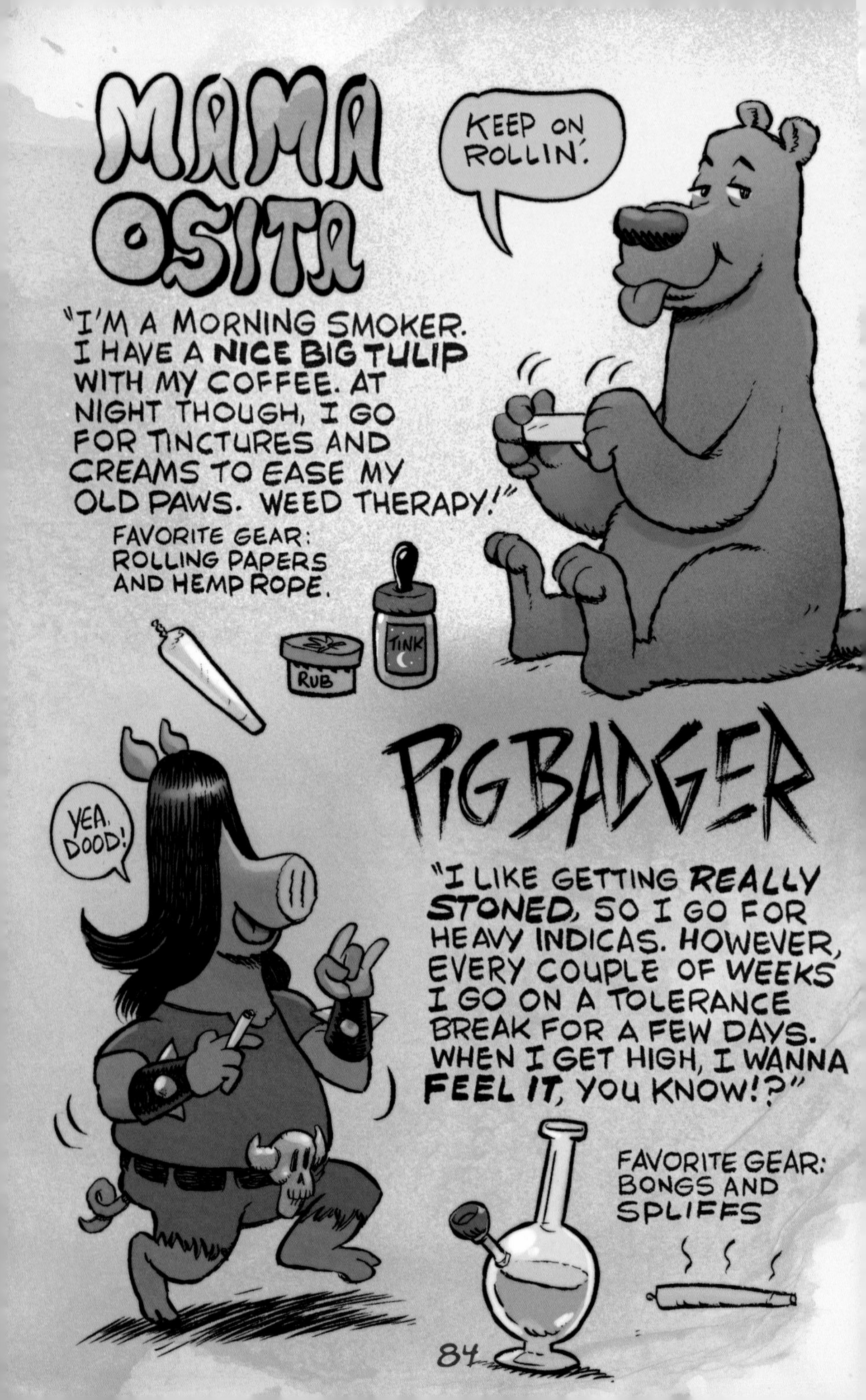
MAMA OSITA
KEEP ON ROLLIN'.
"I'M A MORNING SMOKER. I HAVE A NICE BIG TULIP WITH MY COFFEE. AT NIGHT THOUGH, I GO FOR TINCTURES AND CREAMS TO EASE MY OLD PAWS. WEED THERAPY!"
FAVORITE GEAR: ROLLING PAPERS AND HEMP ROPE.
RUB
TINK
PIGBADGER
YEA, DOOD!
"I LIKE GETTING REALLY STONED, SO I GO FOR HEAVY INDICAS. HOWEVER, EVERY COUPLE OF WEEKS I GO ON A TOLERANCE BREAK FOR A FEW DAYS. WHEN I GET HIGH, I WANNA FEEL IT, YOU KNOW!?"
FAVORITE GEAR: BONGS AND SPLIFFS

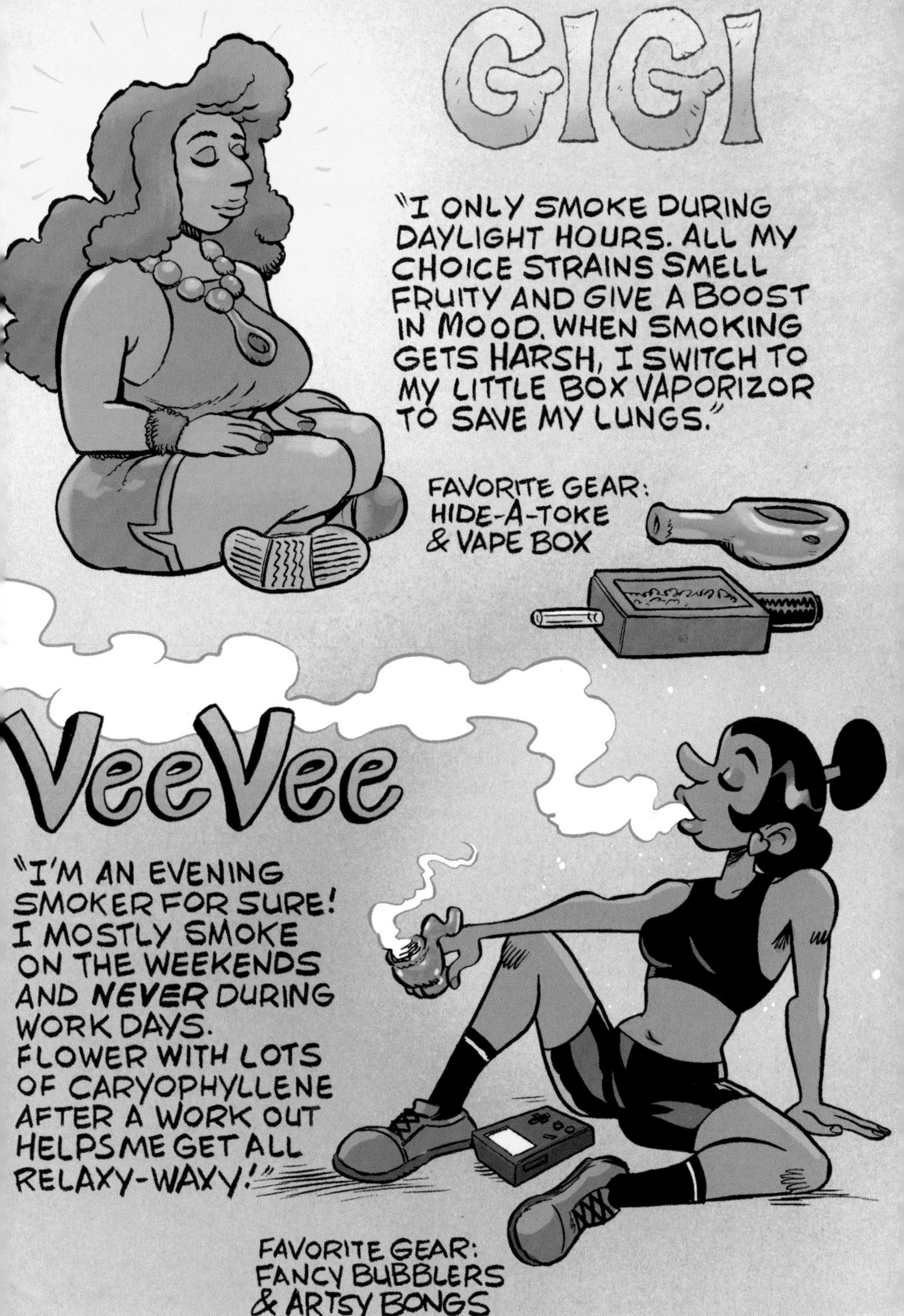
GIGI
"I ONLY SMOKE DURING DAYLIGHT HOURS. ALL MY CHOICE STRAINS SMELL FRUITY AND GIVE A BOOST IN MOOD. WHEN SMOKING GETS HARSH, I SWITCH TO MY LITTLE BOX VAPORIZOR TO SAVE MY LUNGS."
FAVORITE GEAR: HIDE-A-TOKE & VAPE BOX
VeeVee
"I'M AN EVENING SMOKER FOR SURE! I MOSTLY SMOKE ON THE WEEKENDS AND NEVER DURING WORK DAYS. FLOWER WITH LOTS OF CARYOPHYLLENE AFTER A WORK OUT HELPS ME GET ALL RELAXY-WAXY!"
FAVORITE GEAR: FANCY BUBBLERS & ARTSY BONGS

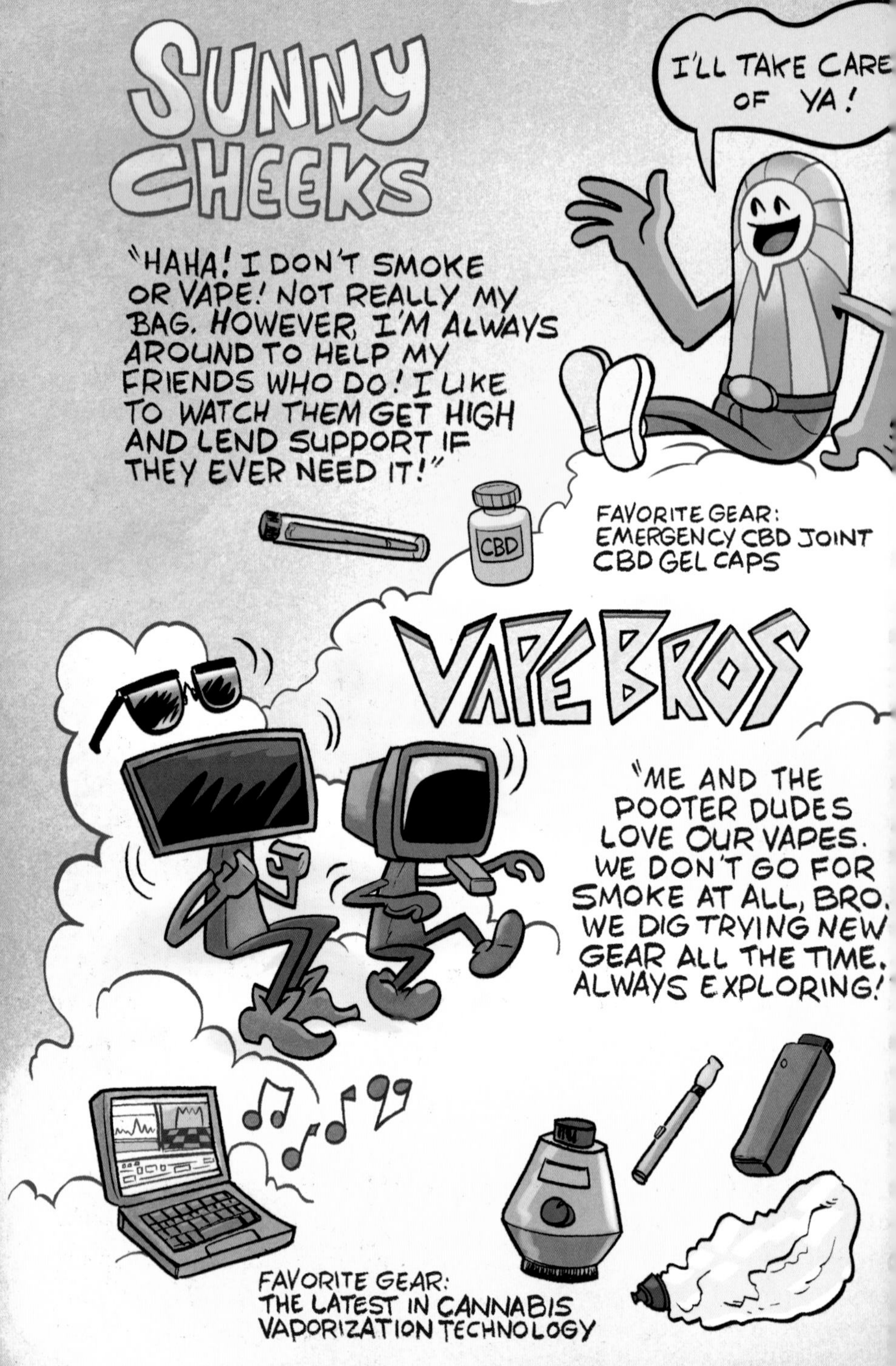
SUNNY CHEEKS
I'LL TAKE CARE OF YA!
"HAHA! I DON'T SMOKE OR VAPE! NOT REALLY MY BAG. HOWEVER, I'M ALWAYS AROUND TO HELP MY FRIENDS WHO DO! I LIKE TO WATCH THEM GET HIGH AND LEND SUPPORT IF THEY EVER NEED IT!"
CBD
FAVORITE GEAR:
EMERGENCY CBD JOINT
CBD GEL CAPS
VAPE BROS
"ME AND THE POOTER DUDES LOVE OUR VAPES. WE DON'T GO FOR SMOKE AT ALL, BRO. WE DIG TRYING NEW GEAR ALL THE TIME. ALWAYS EXPLORING!"
FAVORITE GEAR:
THE LATEST IN CANNABIS VAPORIZATION TECHNOLOGY

GLOSSARY

BAKED: Feeling of being high, but not too high to function while performing activities.

BHO: Butane Hash Oil. A high-potency concentrate. Often called wax or shatter.

BLUNT: Flower wrapped in cigar leaf. These burn for a long time and contain nicotine.

BOGART: Holding a joint too long. Named for actor Humphrey Bogart.

BUD: The flower of the cannabis plant where the THC, CBD, and other compounds are formed.

BUDDER: Concentrate similar to BHO, but softer and more pliable. Very potent.

CHEEBA: Street name for marijuana. "Who wants to smoke a little cheeba?"

CLAMBAKE / HOT BOX: Smoking in an enclosed area like a car or sealed room.

CLONE: Clipping of a plant that can be planted and grown, creating a genetic copy.

CONCENTRATE: Any cannabis that has been refined from flower to a more potent form.

CONE ROLL: A style of large, cone-shaped joint. Sometimes called Dutch tulips.

CROSS-FADING: Getting high while drunk or drunk while high. Can be very dangerous. Not recommended to mix the two.

CRYSTALS: The fine trichomes on the buds of cannabis flowers. Used to make concentrates.

DABS: Slang for highly concentrated THC, like BHO, shatter, or wax.

DANK: Term used to describe very high quality cannabis with strong effects.

DECARBOXYLATION: Heating flower at lower temperatures to activate THCA and CBDA.

DRO: Flower grown indoors in hydroponic chambers. Usually of very high quality.

EIGHTH/HALF/OUNCE: The typical measurements of flower sold.

ENDO: Also called indo. Refers to weed grown indoors, where growers can control conditions.

ENTS: Honorific bestowed upon experienced smokers. "Tree people." Tolkien reference.

GANJA: Word for cannabis flower originated from the Hindi, Urdu, and Sanskrit languages.

GREEN OUT: Akin to "black out". Usually caused by not knowing one's limit for weed.

HEMP: Variety of the cannabis sativa species grown for industrial uses like paper and cloth.

KIEF: Trichomes separated from the cannabis flower through various means.

MOTA: Spanish slang for cannabis. Kind of like weed, Mary Jane, or pot.

SCHWAG: Low-quality flower. Often brown in color, with low THC content and poor flavor.

SHATTER: High-potency concentrated THC. Usually transparent and easily broken up.

SKUNK: Very strong-smelling variety of sativa-dominant hybrid flower.

SPICE: A synthetic marijuana product that is EXTREMELY DANGEROUS. Deaths reported.

TRIM: Remaining leaves cut from cannabis plants after cultivation. Often used to make less expensive concentrates.

TWAX: Process of adding concentrates to your flower via joints or bowls.

TWOMP: Slang for a 20-dollar bag of weed. Refers to the number 20.

VAPORIZATION: A process using moderate heat to produce inhalable vapor from flower or concentrates.

WEED: Dat sticky icky icky, Devil's lettuce, doja, doobage, dope, friendship, ganja, goo, Grandpa's medicine, grass, green, Guy Smiley, herb, jazz cigarette, kine bud, Mary Jane, reefer, silly spinach, trees, wacky tobaccy.

Whatever you like to call it or however you like to take it, always remember: Have respect for this incredible flower and use it responsibly!